ANTICOAGULATION THERAPY

Edited by **Özcan Başaran** and **Murat Biteker**

Anticoagulation Therapy
http://dx.doi.org/10.5772/61447
Edited by Özcan Başaran and Murat Biteker

Contributors

Ozcan Basaran, Volkan Dogan, Ibrahim Altun, Murat Biteker, Ioana Tiuca, Keval Patel, Richard Lee, Ali Mehdirad, Roberto Sant´Anna, Andrey Momot, Lyudmila Tsyvkina, Irina Taranenko, Nadezhda Semenova, Irina Molchanova, Virginie Lattard, Sébastien Lefebvre, Etienne Benoit, Herm Jan Brinkman

Published by InTech

Janeza Trdine 9, 51000 Rijeka, Croatia

Publishing Process Manager Iva Lipovic

Technical Editor SPi Global

Cover InTech Design team

First published September, 2016

Printed in Croatia

Additional hard copies can be obtained from orders@intechopen.com

Anticoagulation Therapy, Edited by Özcan Başaran and Murat Biteker

p. cm.

Print ISBN 978-953-51-2666-9
Online ISBN 978-953-51-2667-6

For EU product safety concerns:
IN TECH d.o.o., Prolaz Marije Krucifikse Kozulić 3, 51000 Rijeka, Croatia,
info@intechopen.com or visit our website at intechopen.com.

Meet the editors

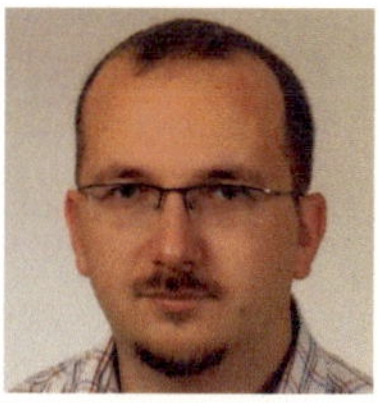

Özcan Başaran is a cardiologist at the Muğla Sıtkı Koçman University Education and Research Hospital. His research interests focus on atrial fibrillation. He has recently conducted ReAl-life Multicenter Survey Evaluating Stroke prevention strategies in Turkey (RAMSES) study. The study aimed to investigate oral anticoagulant use among Turkish atrial fibrillation patients.

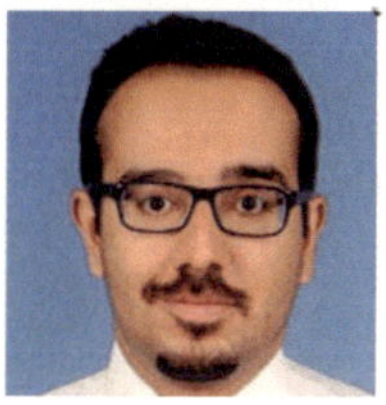

Murat Biteker is associate professor of cardiology at the Muğla Sıtkı Koçman University, Faculty of Medicine. He has published more than 100 international articles. His research interest focuses on valvular heart disease, anticoagulant therapy, peripartum cardiomyopathy, and stroke.

Contents

Preface

Advances in our understanding of the mechanisms of pathogenesis of venous thromboembolism, acute coronary syndromes, cerebral vascular ischemia, and diseases associated with thrombotic events have provided critical insight for the development of various therapeutic approaches to control these pathogenic events. Although numerous parenteral anticoagulants have been available, the vitamin K antagonists have been the only orally active anticoagulant drugs until recently. The last few years have seen the arrival of new drug classes, the orally active direct thrombin inhibitors, and factor Xa antagonists. These drugs do not require frequent monitoring or dose adjustment and have minimal food/drug interactions, but they are not without important drawbacks. Despite their well-documented benefits, anticoagulants continue to be associated with significant morbidity and mortality. *Anticoagulant Therapy* is written in an easy-to-follow format and with many illustrations to aid clarity and assimilation of information. Each chapter is written by established authorities in their fields who are also experienced in explaining often complex concepts. The result is a unique book which is not only comprehensive but also clear and useful for busy medical practitioners. The editors are deeply indebted to the authors for their efforts toward the completion of this comprehensive work.

Özcan Başaran, MD
Cardiology Department,
Muğla Sıtkı Koçman University Education and Research Hospital,
Turkey

Murat Biteker, Associate Professor
Cardiology Department,
Muğla Sıtkı Koçman University Faculty of Medicine,
Turkey

Chapter 1

Biochemistry and Stereochemistry of Anticoagulants

Ioana-Daria Tiuca

Additional information is available at the end of the chapter

http://dx.doi.org/10.5772/64417

Abstract

The spatial conformation of a molecule, in general, is closely connected to its interaction with the human body, meaning bioreceptors, metabolizing enzymes, transporting proteins, etc. This chapter provides useful information regarding the importance of spatial conformation(s) of anticoagulant molecules in their pharmacological activity. It is divided in several sections: firstly, a short introduction is made into the world of stereochemistry, and the importance of this field to the pharmacotherapy is highlighted. Then, each anticoagulant class is treated regarding their spatial orientations and their significance linked to the mechanism of action, anticoagulant activity, potency, etc.

Keywords: stereochemistry, biochemistry, spatial conformation, enantiomer

1. Introduction

The mechanism of action of anticoagulants is very complex, involving many biochemical reactions. The coagulation cascade which is finally blocked and the formation of a clot is stopped in a direct (e.g. direct Xa factor inhibitors) or indirect way (e.g. vitamin K antagonists) assume many reactions, which involve the activation of factors, cofactors and enzymes. The coagulation cascade involves a series of protein conformation changes, which are called "activations" and which are dependent one to each other leading to this cascade series of reactions. Most of these reactions are calcium-dependent, and some of them are vitamin K-dependent (also known as the anti-haemorrhagic vitamin). The coagulation cascade ends with the formation of a fibrin clot, and it can be stopped by interruption by natural ways, such as genetic disorders (e.g. haemophilia A, B or C) or by extrinsic ways, when administering anticoagulants. As well known, when it comes about natural-occurring compounds, these reactions are very specific, but when it comes about external synthetic derivatives, the receptors can be "tricked" in different ways. One cause could be the stereochemistry of these compounds, which is also important for these specific interactions.

Stereochemistry can be named the chemistry of 3D compounds and shows the relationship between a spatial orientation of a molecule and its physical and chemical properties. Very often, when a drug molecule can adopt different spatial shapes and forms, its reactivity with the biomolecules can change. Taking into consideration that from its introduction to the human organism until its excretion, a drug will meet tens, hundreds or even more types of biomolecules, its reactivity is translated into its pharmacological effects, but its toxicity is expected to depend also on its spatial orientation.

The aim of this chapter is to highlight the importance of stereochemistry in anticoagulation therapy, following each subclass of anticoagulants. For this purpose, we present basic notions of stereochemistry with details about the importance of spatial conformations of drug molecules related to the biochemistry of these drugs, and in the end of the chapter, we will find out whether the 3D structure of anticoagulants should be thought of in an anticoagulation treatment plan.

2. Basics of stereochemistry

Stereochemistry is defined as chemistry of spatial isomers. When one refers to stereoisomers, generally they are divided into two categories: firstly, there are the *enantiomers*, which are given by the asymmetry of a certain compound, and secondly, there are the *diastereomers*, which include all other conformational isomers which are not enantiomers.

In living organisms, the isometry given by enantiomers, also called *chirality*, is very important. As mentioned before, they are defined by asymmetry. The asymmetry of a molecule can come in two ways:

- When a carbon atom has four different substituents; in this case, the carbon atom is represented by a centre of asymmetry and is called asymmetrical carbon atom; in this case, one can talk about *planar chirality*; there are other types of atoms, such as N or P, which can confer asymmetry to a molecule, but these cases are rarer.
- Usually, in case of macromolecules, such as polypeptides, proteins, DNA, etc., the whole molecule presents a conformational asymmetry; in this case, one can talk about *intrinsic or helicoidal chirality*. We can say that even the human body, if it were regarded as one molecule, has intrinsic chirality, on the inside and also on the outside, as we are not perfectly symmetrical.

The enantiomers of a molecule are represented as the object and its self-mirror-image (**Figure 1**), which are not superimposable.

Under physical and chemical aspects, the two enantiomers of a pair present the same physical properties (same melting point, same boiling point, same density, etc.) and, unlike diastereomers, have the same chemical properties in non-chiral environment. Their properties differ only in chiral environment.

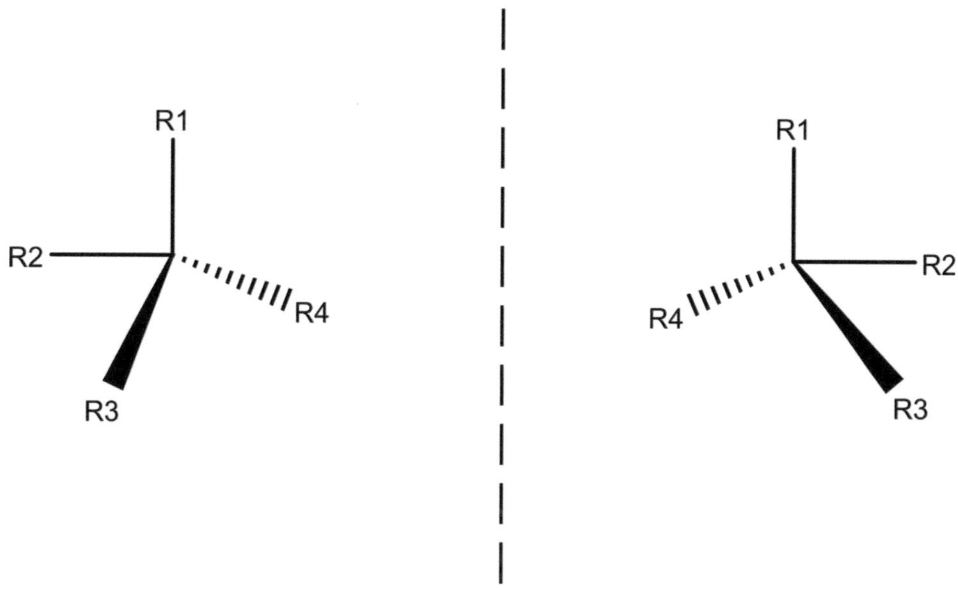

Figure 1. Pair of enantiomers—(S)-enantiomer in the left and (R)-enantiomer in the right—represented as object and its self-mirror-image.

Another different property of enantiomers is their behaviour in polarized light. In one pair of enantiomer, one enantiomer will rotate the plan of polarized light towards the left with a certain angle, while the other one will rotate the plan of polarized light with the same angle but in the other direction. The first enantiomer will be called *levogyre* and is noted (−) or l, and the other one is called *dextrogyre* and is noted (+) or d. The equimolar mixture of the two enantiomers is called *racemic mixture,* is noted with ± and does not affect the plan of polarized light.

Another internationally accepted nomenclature of enantiomers is the Cahn-Ingold-Prelog nomenclature. This uses the absolute configuration of the molecules, which involves the position of the four groups surrounding the asymmetrical carbon atom. They are numbered from the lightest atom directly bonded to the asymmetrical carbon to the heaviest. If the order of reading is towards the right side (or clockwise), the enantiomer is called R (or *rectus*); if the order of reading is towards the left side (or counterclockwise), the enantiomer is called S (or *sinister*) (**Figure 1**). Conventional D or L nomenclature is used for amino acids and saccharides. This should not be confused with the d or l nomenclature. For this reason, to indicate whether an enantiomer is levogyre or dextrogyre, the (+) or (−) notation is preferred.

One molecule will always have a number of 2^{n-1} pairs of enantiomers, where *n* represents the number of centres of asymmetry of the molecule. For example, the coumarinic anticoagulant warfarin (see **Figure 5**) has one centre of asymmetry represented by one asymmetrical carbon atom; thus, the molecule will have two enantiomers or one pair of enantiomers. The optical isomers of the molecule which are not enantiomers (one with each other) are called *diastereomers*. In case of a symmetrical molecule where one chiral centre compensates the effect of another one, the enantiomers are practically identical, and they are called *mesomers*.

There are other types of stereoisomerism, where molecules can adopt different spatial conformations. The conformational isomerism of saccharides is worth mentioning. For example, D-glucose can adopt a chair or a boat conformation, a function of the display of the carbon atoms in the hexa-atomic cycle in space. The helicoidal chirality of proteins and other macromolecules should not be left behind.

2.1. Importance of chirality in human life

The reaction between a drug and its receptor is usually a specific reaction between the target molecule and a protein which acts as receptor. As macromolecules, the protein receptors are almost always chiral, so one can expect in case of chiral drugs to meet an enantioselective drug-receptor interaction, which could lead to different effects translated in the pharmacological activity of the molecule.

When it comes about chiral drugs, there can be five cases in which the two enantiomers of a drug can react with the receptors of the human body, translated in their pharmacological or toxicological activities [1]:

- The most common case is when the two enantiomers have the same pharmacological activities. At first sight, the use of a single enantiomer would not be necessary. However, there are many substances which have one enantiomer (eutomer) 5, 10 up to 60 times more active than the other one (distomer). This is the case of adrenaline, omeprazole or coumarinic anticoagulants. In case of omeprazole, it is long time since the eutomer, (S)-(−)-omeprazole, has been introduced on the pharmaceutical market as the single enantiomer (Nexium®). The case of coumarinic anticoagulants will be discussed in Section 4.

- There can be the case when only one of the enantiomer is pharmacologically active, while the other one is inactive. In this case, a separation of the two enantiomers is not strictly necessary. However, in some cases, when the two enantiomers have different metabolic pathways, a chiral separation could prevent some drug-drug interactions.

- When the eutomer and the distomer have totally opposite pharmacodynamic effects, a chiral separation would be necessary. However, in many cases, the racemic mixture is used in therapy, preserving the effect of the most potent enantiomer.

- Another example is the well-known case of thalidomide, in which the eutomer is responsible for the pharmacological activity, while the distomer is responsible for the adverse effects. In this case, the separation of the two enantiomers is mandatory.

- There are cases when using the racemic mixture is more beneficial, compared to the use of the single enantiomers.

http://dx.doi.org/10.5772/64417

As it can be seen, there are some cases when the use of the single enantiomer in drug therapy is mandatory. Moreover, even in other cases, this choice may have many benefits compared to the classical use of the racemic mixture. For these reasons, some drugs which were previously used as racemic mixtures have been "rediscovered" and have been reintroduced in pharmaceutical formulations as their single enantiomer form. This phenomenon is called *chiral switch*, and one of the most recent examples is represented by dexlansoprazole, the eutomer of lansoprazole, commercialized under the name of Dexilant® [2].

All these above-mentioned indicate clearly that the spatial conformation of an active molecule is very important for its pharmacological activity and, moreover, for its possible toxicological effects to the human body.

3. Heparin and related compounds

Heparin is a natural linear polysaccharide, which belongs to the class of glycosaminoglycans, formed of glucosamine units alternating with glucuronic acid and iduronic acid units, bearing N-sulphate, O-sulphate and N-acetyl groups. It acts as an anticoagulant by binding to antithrombin III and changing its conformation, leading to its activation. It is biosynthesized by enzymatic cleavage of the macromolecular heparin, a proteoglycan. Its composition can be very heterogeneous, depending on the type of tissue where it is extracted from and of the species. A very similar polysaccharidic structure is represented by heparan sulphate.

A specific pentasaccharide sequence (**Figure 2**), formed of glucuronic and iduronic sulphated units, has been identified as the active site of heparin for antithrombin III [3].

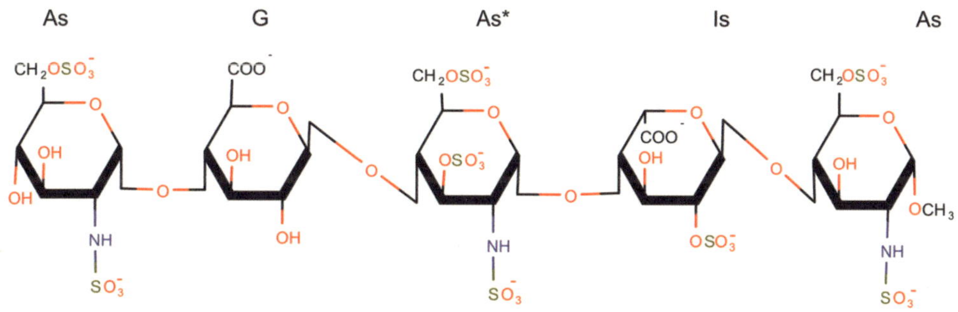

Figure 2. Sequence of the specific pentasaccharide in heparin, which runs as active site for antithrombin III (As, D-glucosamine-N-sulphate; G, α-D-glucuronic acid; As*, D-glucosamine-N-6-disulphate; Is, α-D-iduronic acid).

The conformational studies of the pentasaccharide sequence of heparin realized by ^{1}H-RMN and mechanical calculations [4] have shown that this sequence is formed of a rigid trisaccharide and a more flexible disaccharide. The rigid trisaccharide is based on a glucuronic acid unit, and it is supposed to be responsible for the direct bonding to the active site of antithrombin III, while the flexible disaccharide is based on an iduronic acid unit, it can take several conformations due to the iduronic acid flexibility, which can show different ring conformations, and the "choice" of a certain conformation can decide the bonding to other sites of the antithrombin III molecule. NMR and molecular modelling studies have shown that the iduronate residue in the pentasaccharide sequence can adopt several conformations of the pyranose ring. Results have shown that the most stable conformations in terms of lowest calculated energies are two chair conformations—$^{1}C_4$ and $^{4}C_1$—and a twisted conformation, so-called skew-boat conformation, noted $^{2}S_0$, and in the heparin polymer, the iduronate unit is found as a mixture of these three conformations. Studies have shown these conformations are interconvertible [4–6] (**Figure 3**).

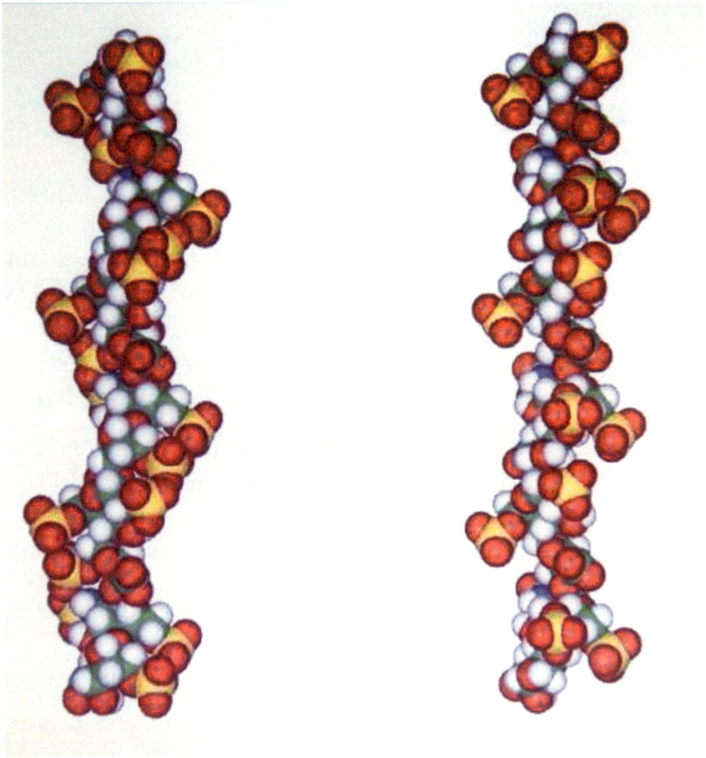

Figure 3. Structures of heparin determined by NMR studies, shown with the iduronic acid unit in the chair $^{1}C_4$ conformation (left) and in the skew-boat $^{2}S_0$ conformation (right). Reproduced from Mulloy and Forster [6] with permission of Oxford University Press.

We can notice that the spatial conformation is very important in case of heparin starting even from its mechanism of action. Jin et al. [7] have elucidated the mechanism of interaction between the heparin-active pentasaccharide and antithrombin III. The mechanistic study revealed that the antithrombin molecule suffers several conformation rearrangements which allow the pentasaccharide to enter the active site. More specific, the α-helix rearranges allowing the formation of hydrogen bonds with the sulphate groups in the pentasaccharide; the α-sheet is closing, while residues in the active loop are partially expulsed, and the D-helix is extended by one-and-a-half turns (**Figure 4**).

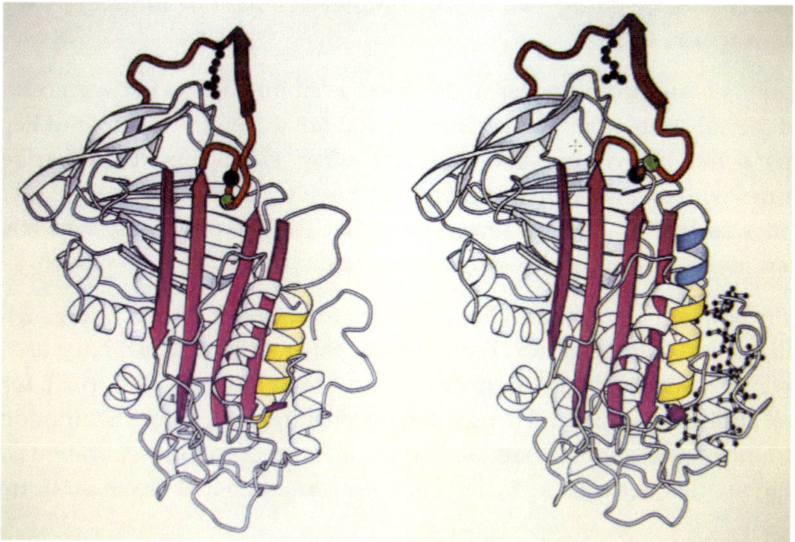

Figure 4. Comparison between free antithrombin III conformation (left) and antithrombin-pentasaccharide complex conformation (right). α-Sheet is closed (magenta), D-helix is extended (blue), and residues in active loop are expulsed (black and green dots). Reproduced from Jin et al. [7] with permission of National Academy of Sciences of the USA.

Thus, the active site loop is partially inserted into the α-sheet, until the antithrombin molecule forms the complex with the pentasaccharide of the heparin polymer. Consequently, the antithrombin-pentasaccharide complex formation and activation model could be extended to the whole heparin polymer. Moreover, by elaborating this model, the authors [7] have demonstrated the importance of conformation changes which take place in antithrombin molecule. A valuable example is the case of natural mutations of antithrombin, which lead to thromboembolic syndrome. Any replacement of any amino acid in the active site of the antithrombin molecule will lead to its inactivity by incapacity of conformation change, because of incomplete or lack of binding sites to the pentasaccharide.

In addition to the conformational change of antithrombin, Verli and Guimarães [8] have described the conformational change of the pentasaccharide, when forming the complex with antithrombin, thus leading to an induced fit mechanism of reaction. A change in the dihedral angles between the glucosamine and iduronic acid unit and, respectively, between glucosamine and glucuronic acid unit, from 20 to 30° was observed, even if the pentasaccharide was in skew-boat $^2S_0$ conformation or in chair $^1C_4$ conformation. This gives a new perspective to the mechanism of interaction between heparin and antithrombin, where the conformational flexibility is important on both sides, the ligand and the substrate. Taking a deeper view into the induced fit mechanism of interaction between heparin and antithrombin, it is worth mentioning that there is a need of 7 up to 30 hydrogen bonds for the complex to get formed. This information is essential for the drug development and design for new anticoagulant structures, heparin-related [8]. For example, the highly sulphated saccharidic polymer of heparin was replaced by a highly sulphated lignin, to obtain a new anticoagulant potential drug [9], with reduced bleeding side effects compared to the low-molecular-weight heparin derivative, enoxaparin.

As the activation of antithrombin was understood as an interaction between certain oligosaccharides and the substrate, thus understanding that not the entire polymer of heparin participates in the activation of the antithrombin, other similar pentasaccharides or other oligosaccharides with potential anticoagulant activity have also been synthesized. In the same time, heparin was fractionated to lower-molecular-weight polymers, which were not as heterogeneous in composition as the original heparin.

The chirality (asymmetry) of heparin has also been used in chiral separations, where heparin has been utilized as a chiral selector. For example, Jin and Stalcup [10] have used heparin as chiral additive to the background electrolyte in capillary electrophoresis (CE), for the separation of several antihistaminic chiral drugs, such as pheniramine, chlorpheniramine, brompheniramine, carbinoxamine and doxylamine. The mechanism of enantioseparation was proposed as being a combination between inclusion complex formation and electrostatic interaction.

4. Coumarinic anticoagulants (vitamin K antagonists)

Unlike heparin and related derivatives, coumarinic anticoagulants have relatively small molecules, and their anticoagulant mechanism of action is totally different. They act by inhibiting the epoxide reductase which is involved in the recovery of vitamin K, after its oxidation.

Warfarin is the most prescribed coumarinic anticoagulant in the USA and UK. Besides warfarin, in other European countries, acenocoumarol and phenprocoumon are used as vitamin K antagonists (**Figure 5**). In all three cases, they present chiral structures as they contain a chiral carbon atom in their molecule, leading to the existence of two enantiomers in each case.

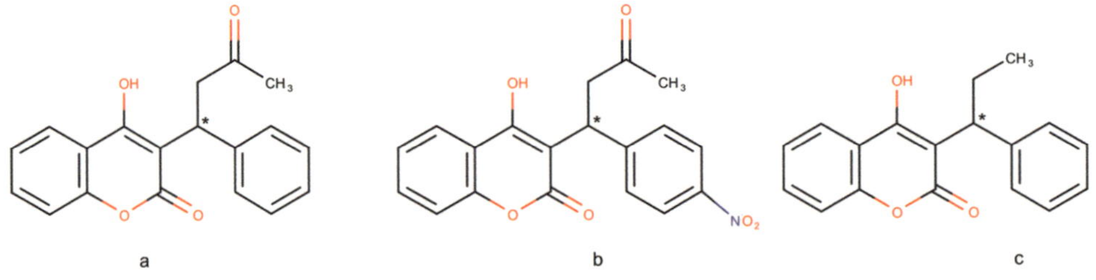

Figure 5. Molecular structures of coumarinic anticoagulants: (a) warfarin, (b) acenocoumarol, and (c) phenprocoumon; chiral centre is indicated with asterisk (C*).

In all three cases, there is a difference in the anticoagulant activity between the two enantiomers of the substance. In case of warfarin and phenprocoumon, their (S)-(−)-enantiomers are two up to five times more active than their optical isomers, (R)-(+)-phenprocoumon, and (R)-(+)-

warfarin, respectively. In case of acenocoumarol, the (R)-(+)-antipode is around five times more active than the (S)-(−)-enantiomer [11].

It is worth mentioning that the difference of only one nitro group between warfarin and acenocoumarol structures leads to the reversal of potency of anticoagulant activity between the two enantiomers; in consequence, (R)-(+)-warfarin and (S)-(−)-acenocoumarol are the more potent ones.

This difference of anticoagulant activity between the enantiomers of coumarinic anticoagulants comes from two directions. Firstly, there are the genetic determinants, and secondly, the different metabolic pathways can explain these differences.

To understand the two types of differences, one should understand the mechanism of action of these anticoagulants. Briefly, they act by interfering in vitamin K-dependent reactions in the organism [11]. Vitamin K, also known as coagulation vitamin or anti-haemorrhagic vitamin, is required for the liver synthesis of some coagulation factors (II, VII, IX and X), protein C and protein S. On the one hand, the above-mentioned molecules become active in γ-carboxylation reaction vitamin K-dependent. Inactive proteins cannot pass through the coagulation cascade. On the other hand, during these reactions, vitamin K suffers an oxidation to a 2,3-epoxide form, which is inactive. The vitamin K 2,3-epoxide reductase (VKOR) is the enzyme which brings vitamin K to its initial active form.

The coumarinic anticoagulants act by inhibiting the 2,3-epoxide reductase. Consequently, vitamin K remains inactive, and so factors II, VII, IX and X remain inactive, and the coagulation cascade is stopped.

Several studies [12–15] reveal that the main genetic polymorphisms responsible for the inter-patient variability are for the VKOR enzyme, under its different VKORC1 haplotypes and the cytochrome P450 2C9 isoenzyme (CYP2C9), involved in the metabolism of these coumarinic anticoagulants. However, a more recent study [16] has proven the significant relationship between VKORC1 genotypes and differences in pharmacodynamics of warfarin enantiomers. The authors have shown that patients with TT genotype of VKORC1 are more sensitive to (S)-warfarin and relatively more sensitive to (R)-warfarin. They have proven a clear anticoagulant contribution of (R)-(+)-warfarin to the racemic mixture, even if the (S)-warfarin is the more potent one. However, when administering the racemic in polytherapy, drug-drug interactions may also occur because of (R)-warfarin; likewise, when administering an inhibitor of (R)-warfarin, such as cimetidine, an increase in the anticoagulant effect is likely to appear. As these interactions do not appear in all populations, it is likely to notice a relationship between (R)-warfarin contribution to drug-drug interactions and the VKORC1 genotype [16].

The genotypes of the CYP2C9 isoenzyme are closely related to the anticoagulant activity of these three molecules and their enantiomers. As this isoenzyme of CYP450 is the main route of metabolism for all three drugs, there is a very close relationship between the pharmacogenetics, pharmacokinetics and in the end pharmacodynamics of the molecule. Thijssen and Ritzen [17] have proven the influence of CYP2C9 polymorphism on the different pharmacokinetics of the two enantiomers of acenocoumarol. The study results revealed that the plasma concentrations of (S)-acenocoumarol at 7 hours after administration of racemic were higher for patients who presented the CYP2C9*2 or CYP2C9*3 alleles, compared to the control group of CYP2C9*1/*1. In contrast, for (R)-acenocoumarol, it was not observed any significant influence of the CYP2C9 polymorphism over its plasma concentration, when determined at 7 hours or at 24 hours after administration. For (S)-acenocoumarol, the plasma concentration at 24 hours was not detectable (see **Table 1**). These results show the importance of optical conformation of a drug in vivo. In addition to all these data, in some cases, the presence of other CYP2C9 alleles, such as *4, *5 or *6, should be taken in consideration [17]. In case of warfarin and phenprocoumon, there is not such a distinct difference of clearance between the two enantiomers, as can be seen in **Figure 6**.

Genotype	(S)-acenocoumarol (ng/mL)		(R)-acenocoumarol (ng/mL)		
	4 hours after intake	7 hours after intake	4 hours after intake	7 hours after intake	24 hours after intake
*1/*1 (n = 9)	34.9 ± 18.1	5.1 ± 4.2	219 ± 48	146 ± 21	34.5 ± 5.3
*1/*2 (n = 7)	26.3 ± 12.5	9.9 ± 4.9	199 ± 40	135 ± 31	31.7 ± 5.9
*1/*3 (n = 6)	47.7 ± 18.7	14.6 ± 6.6	226 ± 31	151 ± 35	30.7 ± 16.9
*2/*3 (n = 3)	33.2 ± 8.0	16.6 ± 5.0	163 ± 27	136 ± 36	33.9 ± 0.6
*2/*2 (n = 1)	59.6	25.8	180	167	ND

ND, not determined; *n*, number of patients. Reproduced from Thijssen and Ritzen [17] with permission of John Wiley and Sons, Inc.

Table 1. Plasma (R)- and (S)-acenocoumarol concentrations after oral intake of 8 mg racemic acenocoumarol: effect of CYP2C9 polymorphism.

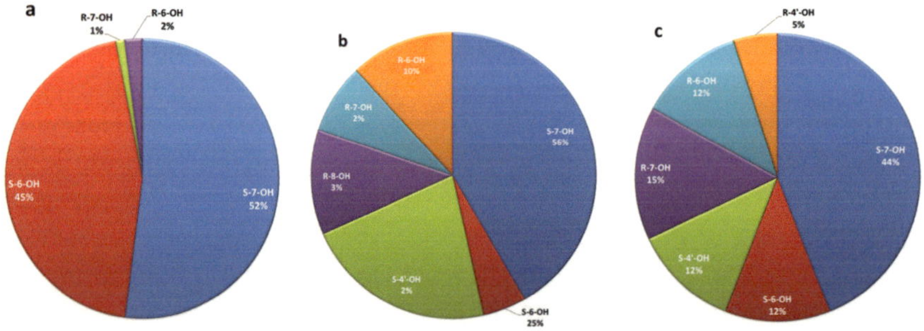

Figure 6. Intrinsic clearances of (a) (S)-acenocoumarol and (R)-acenocoumarol, (b) (S)-warfarin and (R)-warfarin and (c) (S)-phenprocoumon and (R)-phenprocoumon, as calculated from Thijssen et al. [18, 19] and Ufer et al. [20].

As could be seen, the genetic polymorphism leads to a difference in pharmacokinetics of the two enantiomers. In case of acenocoumarol, as it can be seen in **Table 1**, the half-life of (S)-enantiomer is much shorter than of the (R)-enantiomer. In case of CYP2C9*1/*3, the half-life of (S)-acenocoumarol may be even doubled, up to 4 hours, which may lead to an increase in anticoagulant activity. However, even if (S)-acenocoumarol is one of the most potent anticoagulants in the 4-hydroxycoumarin class [18], its half-life seems to be too short for the (S)-acenocoumarol to interfere in the vitamin K-dependent reactions and to stop the coagulation cascade. Consequently, we can say that generally the effect of the racemic mixture is given by the (R)-acenocoumarol.

Another difference of pharmacokinetics between the two acenocoumarol enantiomers is given by the isoenzymes responsible for their metabolism. While CYP2C9 [18] seems to be the main enzyme to transform (S)-acenocoumarol to its 6- and 7-hydroxy-metabolites, in case of (R)-acenocoumarol, there are several enzymes involved in this process, which can explain the difference in their resulting in vivo half-life. (R)-acenocoumarol is 7-hydroxylated by CYP2C9, but the 6-hydroxylation is mediated, partially by other CYP450 isoenzymes, such as CYP1A2 and CYP2C19. For these enzymes, other drug-drug interactions in polytherapy cases should be predicted.

Phenprocoumon [12] seems to be less affected by CYP2C9, but its metabolism is realized mainly by CYP3A4. Moreover, a significant quantity of this anticoagulant is eliminated under untransformed form, while acenocoumarol and warfarin are almost totally metabolized through hydroxylation. CYP4F2 and CYP2C18 have also been mentioned to participate in the metabolism of coumarinic anticoagulants. Genetic polymorphism should be taken in consideration in this case, too. At the same time, different genetic variants of enzymes involved in the chain of reactions on which the anticoagulant mechanism of these molecules is based should be considered. For example, the different genotypes of epoxide-hydrolase (EPHX1) and γ-glutamyl carboxylase (GGCX) can lead to different anticoagulant potencies [20–22].

Taking all these in consideration, it remains one question: is it worth to introduce the single enantiomer use in therapy for these drugs? The answer is that in all cases, it should at least be reflected about. The different routes of metabolism for the two pair-enantiomers, influenced partially by pharmacogenetic factors as seen, give them not only different half-lives but also different anticoagulant potencies. In addition to these, one should consider that in most cases, these drugs come in polytherapy, exposing the patient to many drug-drug interactions. When eliminating one of the two enantiomers, at least some of these metabolic pathways which lead to drug-drug interactions can be eliminated. In this case, also food-drug interactions should be considered, which can be partially eliminated, and by reducing the dose, the toxicity and probably some of the adverse effects should decrease. So, as in other drug cases (e.g. omeprazole and lansoprazole), a chiral switch may be considered for these coumarinic anticoagulants. However, in case of acenocoumarol, even if the most anticoagulant active enantiomer seems to be (S)-acenocoumarol, its short half-life makes it almost unusable, while the other enantiomer, (R)-acenocoumarol, which could be kept, presents many metabolic pathways which anyways could not be avoided. In this case, other factors, such as economic elements, may be considered, when having a chiral separation or chiral synthesis for the single enantiomer use.

There have been numerous chiral separation methods developed for the separation of these three chiral drugs. These separations can be realized by high-performance liquid chromatography (HPLC), coupled with UV [23, 24] or mass spectrometer (MS) [25] detectors or by capillary electrophoresis (CE) [26, 27]. However, in case of drug control analysis or chiral purity analysis, there is not necessarily the need to effectively separate the two enantiomers but to know the enantiomeric ratio. For this purpose, p-tert-butylcalix[6]arene derivative has been used as chiral selector for the chiral enantiorecognition of warfarin [28] in a UV-spectral study coupled with the multivariate analysis of the spectral data. The results showed a good capacity of enantiorecognition of the achiral molecule of calixarene towards the enantiomers of warfarin, being able to determine the ratio of one enantiomer when this was in a proportion of up to 5 % in the mixture. The impact of this study relies not only in the determination of the enantiomeric ratio but in the fact that with the aid of multivariate analysis, which can interpret seemingly messy and complicated data, the different behaviour of enantiomers can be discovered even in achiral media, as achiral structures were used as chiral selectors.

5. Direct Xa factor and thrombin inhibitors

As this type of anticoagulants represents recently discovered molecules, their chirality has been already explored in the preclinical phase studies, as regulators in the field (Food and Drug Administration) demand it. To highlight once again the importance of chirality in medical and pharmacological field, it is worth mentioning that among these substances, all which are chiral, are used under their single enantiomer form (**Figure 7**).

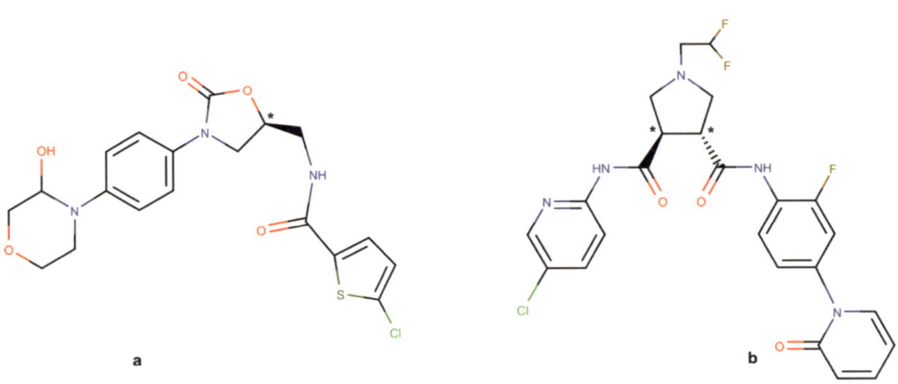

Figure 7. Molecular structures of some direct Xa factor inhibitors: (a) rivaroxaban and (b) R1663, with indication of chiral centre(s).

For example, the (S)-enantiomer of rivaroxaban is used in therapy, as it has a 10,000 times higher affinity towards the active site of Xa factor compared to its pair enantiomer or its diastereomers [29]. In contrast, the (R,R)-enantiomer of otamixaban is preferred as anticoagulant agent [30] as it fits better into the active site of Xa factor. In a similar way, the (R,R)-enantiomer of a novel molecule, (3R,4R)-1-(2,2-difluoro-ethyl)-pyrrolidine-3,4-dicarboxylic acid 3-[(5-chloro-pyridin-2-yl)-amide] 4-{[2-fluoro-4-(2-oxo-2H-pyridin-1-yl)-phenyl]-amide}, named R1663, has already passed phase 1 clinical study for its introduction on the drug market [31]. Edoxaban is another inhibitor of Xa factor used as the single enantiomer in therapy, while it has three asymmetrical carbon atoms in its molecule.

All these differences in spatial conformation actually exhibit a higher anticoagulant potency or activity by a better interaction with the active site of the target substrate. The interaction with the Xa factor must be seen like a "hand-glove" acceptance, where only one "hand" is most suitable for the "glove".

In a similar way, in case of chiral molecules used in therapy as thrombin inhibitors, one should expect to see a difference in affinity towards the substrate, with a higher anticoagulant activity of one enantiomer compared to the other one. Thus, the thrombin inhibitor argatroban (**Figure 8**) is used in its single enantiomer form as (R,R)-enantiomer [32].

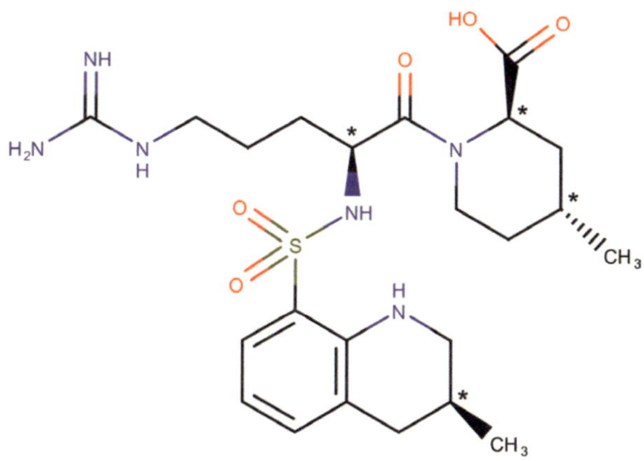

Figure 8. Molecular chiral structure of argatroban, with indication of all chiral centres (C*).

6. Proteic anticoagulants

Proteins, by their nature of macromolecules, are very dependent on their spatial conformation. All natural proteins and polypeptides are formed of natural L-amino acids. The spatial conformation of proteins is crucial for their activity as enzymes, drug receptors, etc.

Thrombin and antithrombin, as it could be seen previously, are two proteins involved in the cascade of coagulation. There are several polypeptidic and proteic anticoagulants used in therapy, which generally target these two molecules. It is worth mentioning the first introduction in therapy, in 2009, of recombinant human antithrombin-α obtained from transgenic goats' milk [33].

Another protein that has given very good results as anticoagulant in deep vein thrombosis is batroxobin, a toxin extracted from *Bothrops atrox* and *Bothrops moojeni* venom [34]. Results showed successful limb salvage for all patients taken in study after they were administered batroxobin, due to anticoagulant and fibrinolytic mechanism of this molecule.

Hirudin is an antithrombin-like protein which possesses anticoagulant effects. It is a smaller proteic molecule which binds to thrombin into its active site. Mengwasser et al. [35] have studied the hirudin-thrombin complex, in terms of stability, affinity one to each other and conformation. Results showed a higher affinity of hirudin towards the fast (F) allosteric form of thrombin, compared to the slow (S) form. There are common residues responsible for both complex formations, but there are seven residues which are responsible for the more than 10 times higher affinity of hirudin towards the F form of thrombin. The residues Asp221 and Asp222 do not interact directly with hirudin, the effect being probably a stabilization of the S form by Na^{+} binding. The same effect could be for Gly-193. The other four residues—Lys36, Leu65, Thr74 and Arg75—do interact directly with hirudin. The preference towards the F form stays probably due to the different spatial orientation of these residues, leading to a better "match" with hirudin in the F form (**Figure 9**).

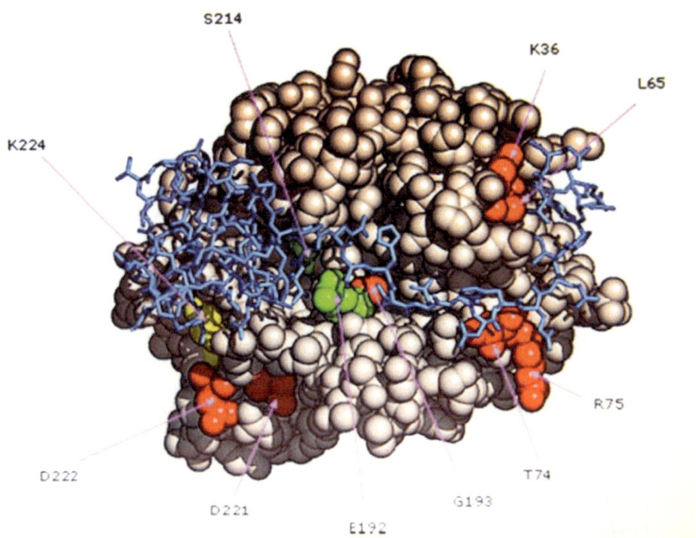

Figure 9. Model of binding of hirudin (marine sticks) to the F (red) and S (green) forms of thrombin. The higher affinity of hirudin towards F thrombin is indicated through the seven residues. The important residue Lys224, which makes an important contribution to hirudin binding, is spotted in yellow. Reproduced from Mengwasser et al. [35] with permission of the American Society for Biochemistry and Molecular Biology.

7. Concluding remarks

Taking all the above-mentioned in consideration, one can say that stereochemistry and the spatial conformations play a key role in the life of a drug molecule, in general, and of an anticoagulant, in special, in terms of pharmacogenetics, pharmacokinetics, pharmacotoxicology and/or pharmacodynamics. When talking about macromolecules, we cannot separate them from their spatial conformation, which is an essential factor which influences their activity. In case of small molecules, the existence of one or more pairs of enantiomers gives them the possibility to act differently with the chiral receptors of the organism, with possible different effects to be observed. As already seen, these reactions depend also on the flexibility of both the target molecule and the receptor macromolecule, but they usually take place following a "hand-glove" model. Stereochemistry of anticoagulants is important in all aspects and should be considered before establishing a treatment plan.

Acknowledgements

The authors are grateful for the financial support from the Romanian National Authority for Scientific Research UEFISCDI for project no. PN-II-RU-TE-2014-4-0460.

Author details

Ioana-Daria Tiuca

Address all correspondence to: tiuca.daria@umfcluj.ro

"Iuliu Haţieganu" University of Medicine and Pharmacy, Cluj-Napoca, Romania

References

[1] Zhang J, Lin G. Chiral drugs and associated asymmetric synthesis. In: Huang Z, editor. Drug Discovery Research: New Frontiers in the Post-Genomic Era. San Diego: Wiley Interscience; 2007. p. 230–78.

[2] Gellad WF, Choi P, Mizah M, Good CB, Kesselheim AS. Assessing the chiral switch: Approval and use of single-enantiomer drugs, 2001 to 2011. Am J Manag Care. 2014;20(3):90–7.

[3] Casu B. Heparin structure. Haemostasis. 1990;20(suppl 1):62–73. DOI: 10.1159/000216162

[4] Ragazzi M, Ferro D, Perly B, Sinay P, Petitou M, Choay J. Conformation of the pentasaccharide corresponding the binding site of heparin for antithrombin III. Carbohydr Res. 1990;195(2):169–85. DOI:10.1016/0008-6215(90)84165-Q

[5] Mulloy B, Forster MJ, Jones C, Davies DB. N.m.r. and molecular-modelling studies of the solution conformation of heparin. Biochem J. 1993;293(3):849–58. DOI: 10.1042/bj2930849

[6] Mulloy B, Forster MJ. Conformation and dynamics of heparin and heparan sulfate. Glycobiology. 2000;10(11):1147–56. DOI: 10.1093/glycob/10.11.1147

[7] Jin L, Abrahams JP, Skinner R, Petitou M, Pike RM, Carrell RW. The anticoagulant activation of antithrombin by heparin. Proc Natl Acad Sci USA. 1997;94(26):14683–8.

[8] Verli H, Guimarães JA. Insights into the induced fit mechanism in antithrombin - heparin interaction using molecular dynamics simulations. J Mol Graph Model. 2005;24(3):203–12. DOI: 10.1016/j.jmgm.2005.07.002

[9] Mehta AY, Mohammed BM, Martin EJ, Brophy DF, Gailani D, Desai UR. Allosterism-based simultaneous, dual anticoagulant and antiplatelet action: Allosteric inhibitor targeting the glycoprotein Ib ?-binding and heparin-binding site of thrombin. J Thromb Haemost. 2016; 14(4):828–38. DOI: 10.1111/jth.13254

[10] Jin Y, Stalcup AM. Application of heparin to chiral separations of antihistamines by capillary electrophoresis. Electrophoresis. 2000;19(12):2119–23. DOI: 10.1002/elps.1150191213

[11] Hirsh J, Fuster V, Ansell J, Halperin JL. American Heart Association/American College of Cardiology foundation guide to warfarin therapy. J Am Coll Cardiol. 2003;41(9):1633–52. DOI: 10.1016/S0735-1097(03)00416-9.

[12] Cadamuro J, Dieplinger B, Felder T, Kedenko I, Mueller T, Haltmayer M et al. Genetic determinants of acenocoumarol and phenprocoumon maintenance dose requirements. Eur J Clin Pharmacol. 2010;66(3):253–60. DOI: 10.1007/s00228-009-0768-7.

[13] Schwarz UI, Ritchie MD, Bradford Y, Li C, Dudek SM, Frye-Anderson A et al. Genetic determinants of response to warfarin during initial anticoagulation. N Engl J Med. 2008;358(10):999–1008. DOI: 10.1056/NEJMoa0708078

[14] Sconce EA, Khan TI, Wynne HA, Avery P, Monkhouse L, Barry P et al. The impact of CYP2C9 and VKORC1 genetic polymorphism and patient characteristics upon warfarin dose requirements: Proposal for a new dosing regimen Blood. 2005;106(7):2329–33. DOI: 10.1182/blood-2005-03-1108.

[15] Manolopoulos VG, Ragia G, Tavridou A. Pharmacogenetics of coumarinic oral anticoagulants. Pharmacogenomics. 2010;11(4):493–6. DOI: 10.2217/pgs.10.31.

[16] Maddison J, Somogyi AA, Jensen BP, James HM, Gentgall M, Rolan PE. The pharmacokinetics and pharmacodynamics of single dose (R)- and (S)-warfarin administered separately and together: Relationship to VKORC1 genotype. Br J Clin Pharmacol. 2013;75(1):208–16. DOI: 10.1111/j.1365-2125.2012.04335.x.

[17] Thijssen HHW, Ritzen B. Acenocoumarol pharmacokinetics in relation to cytochrome P450 2C9 genotype. Clin Pharmacol. Ther 2003;74(1):61–8. DOI: 10.1016/S0009-9236(03)00088-2.

[18] Thijssen HH, Flinois JP, Beaune PH. Cytochrome P4502C9 is the principal catalyst of racemic acenocoumarol hydroxylation reactions in human liver microsomes. Drug Metab Dispos. 2000;28(11):1284–90.

[19] Hermans JJ, Thijssen HH. Human liver microsomal metabolism of the enantiomers of warfarin and acenocoumarol: P450 isozyme diversity determines the differences in their pharmacokinetics. Br J Pharmacol. 1993;110(1):482–90. DOI: 10.1111/j.1476-5381.1993.tb13836.x.

[20] Ufer M, Svensson JO, Krausz KW, Gelboin H V., Rane A, Tybring G. Identification of cytochromes P450 2C9 and 3A4 as the major catalysts of phenprocoumon hydroxylation in vitro. Eur J Clin Pharmacol. 2004;60(3):173–82. DOI: 10.1007/s00228-004-0740-5.

[21] Pautas E, Moreau C, Gouin-Thibault I, Golmard JL, Mahe I, Legendre C et al. Genetic factors (VKORC1, CYP2C9, EPHX1, and CYP4F2) are predictor variables for warfarin response in very elderly, frail inpatients. Clin Pharmacol Ther. 2010;87(1):57–64. DOI: 10.1038/clpt.2009.178.

[22] Teichert M, Eijgelsheim M, Rivadeneira F, Uitterlinden AG, van Schaik RHN, Hofman A et al. A genome-wide association study of acenocoumarol maintenance dosage. Hum Mol Genet. 2009;18(19):3758–68. DOI: 10.1093/hmg/ddp309.

[23] Ding GS, Huang XJ, Liu Y, Wang JD. Chiral separation of racemates of drugs and amino acid derivatives by high-performance liquid chromatography on a norvancomycin-bonded chiral stationary phase. Chromatographia. 2004;(7):443–9. DOI: 10.1365/s10337-004-190-3.

[24] Valliappan K, Vaithiyanathan SJ, Palanivel V. Direct chiral HPLC method for the simultaneous determination of warfarin enantiomers and its impurities in raw material and pharmaceutical formulation: Application of chemometric protocol. Chromatographia. 2013;76(5–6):287–92. DOI: 10.1007/s10337-012-2373-7.

[25] Jensen BP, Chin PKL, Begg EJ. Quantification of total and free concentrations of R- and S-warfarin in human plasma by ultrafiltration and LC-MS/MS. Anal Bioanal Chem. 2011;401(7):2187–93. DOI: 10.1007/s00216-011-5303-x

[26] Chankvetadze B, Burjanadze N, Crommen J, Blaschke G. Enantioseparation of warfarin by capillary electrophoresis with UV and LIF detection using single and dual cyclodextrin type chiral selectors. Chromatographia. 2001;53(suppl1):296–301. DOI: 10.1007/BF02490345

[27] Nowak P, Garnysz M, Mitoraj MP, Sagan F, Wo?niakiewicz M, Ko?cielniak P. Analytical aspects of achiral and cyclodextrin-mediated capillary electrophoresis of warfarin and its two main derivatives assisted by theoretical modeling. J Chromatogr A. 2015;1377:106–13. DOI: 10.1016/j.chroma.2014.12.030

[28] Bodoki E, Tiuca I, Iacob BC, Hosu O, Oprean R. Determination of the enantiomeric ratio of warfarin in tablets by multivariate calibration and modeling of spectroscopic data. Farmacia. 2012;60(3):386–93.

[29] Roehrig S, Straub A, Pohlmann J, Lampe T, Pernerstorfer J, Schlemmer K-H et al. Discovery of the novel antithrombotic agent 5-chloro-N-({(5S)-2-oxo-3-[4-(3-oxomorpholin-4-yl)phenyl]-1,3-oxazolidin-5-yl}methyl)thiophene-2-carboxamide

(BAY59-7939): An oral, direct factor Xa inhibitor. J Med Chem. 2005;48(19):5900–8. DOI: 18 10.1021/jm050101d.

[30] Guertin KR, Choi Y-M. The discovery of the Factor Xa inhibitor otamixaban: From lead identification to clinical development. Curr Med Chem. 2007;14(23):2471–81. DOI: 10.2174/092986707782023659.

[31] Anselm L, Banner DW, Benz J, Groebke Zbinden K, Himber J, Hilpert H et al. Discovery of a factor Xa inhibitor (3R,4R)-1-(2,2-difluoro-ethyl)- pyrrolidine-3,4-dicarboxylic acid 3-[(5-chloro-pyridin-2-yl)-amide] 4-{[2-fluoro-4-(2-oxo-2H-pyridin-1-yl)-phenyl]-amide} as a clinical candidate. Bioorganic Med Chem Lett. 2010;20(17):5313–9. DOI: 10.1016/j.bmcl.2010.06.126.

[32] Ferraboschi P, Mieri M De, Grisenti P, Lotz M, Nettekoven U. Diastereoselective synthesis of an argatroban intermediate, ethyl (2R,4R)-4-methylpipecolate, by means of a Mandyphos/rhodium complex-catalyzed hydrogenation. Tetrahedron Asymmetry. 2011;22(16–17):1626–31. DOI: 10.1016/j.tetasy.2011.09.009

[33] Kling J. First US approval for a transgenic animal drug. Nat Biotechnol. 2009;27(4):302–4. DOI: 10.1038/nbt0409-302

[34] Zhang L, Lu SH, Li L, Tao YG, Wan YL, Senga H et al. Batroxobin mobilizes circulating endothelial progenitor cells in patients with deep vein thrombosis. Clin Appl Thromb Hemost. 2011;17(1):75–9. DOI: 10.1177/1076029609347903.

[35] Mengwasser KE, Bush LA, Shih P, Cantwell AM, Di Cera E. Hirudin binding reveals key determinants of thrombin allostery. J Biol Chem. 2005;280(29):26997–7003. DOI: 10.1074/jbc.M502678200

Comparative Biology of the Resistance to Vitamin K Antagonists: An Overview of the Resistance Mechanisms

Sébastien Lefebvre, Etienne Benoit and
Virginie Lattard

Additional information is available at the end of the chapter

http://dx.doi.org/10.5772/64204

Abstract

Vitamin K antagonists (VKA) are used in human medicine as well as for the management of rodent populations. In both cases, we have to deal with inter-individual resistances. Many mechanisms of resistances are common in humans and rodents. Moreover, with the large use of vitamin K antagonist rodenticides, the resistant phenotype is overrepresented in some rodent populations. Consequently, some resistance mechanisms with a low prevalence in the human population have a higher prevalence in rodent population; thus, they can be more studied in rodents. The aim of this chapter is to cross knowledge coming from human medicine and rodent research in order to better understand each resistance mechanism. After an overview of the essential knowledge for the understanding of the VKA action, this chapter presents the different methods of VKA resistance studying and then it assesses the current knowledge on VKA resistance in humans and rodents.

Keywords: vitamin K antagonists, warfarin, comparative biology, pharmacogenomics

1. Introduction

Vitamin K antagonists (VKA) are inhibitors of the regeneration cycle of vitamin K. The diminution of the available and usable vitamin K in the body induced by VKA leads indirectly to a hypocoagulable status of the blood. The use of VKA in humans and rodents pursues this status. Nevertheless, the final aim is different for each. In the human case, VKA anticoagulants are used to prevent venous and arterial thrombotic event. In spite of the increasing use of new oral anticoagulants, VKA and, more precisely, warfarin are the most commonly prescribed anticoagulants [1]. Considering rodents, VKA are used in pest population management. In this case, death resulting from hemorrhages is pursued. VKA are currently the most used and one of the best rodenticides for two reasons. First, the delay between VKA administration and death is of several days, which avoids association between bait and death by the other rodents. Second, conversely to other rodenticides, VKA have an antidote: the vitamin K, which increases their safety for the human population and nontarget species.

In humans, VKA anticoagulants have a narrow therapeutic range [2]. Under- and overdoses can have serious consequences by the lack of efficacy or adverse event. Warfarin has been ranked number 9 among primary suspect drugs having serious outcomes in the United States during the beginning of the 2000's decade [3]. Indeed, the VKA dose has to be modulated, reflecting the genotype of patients more than other common drugs. Thus, it is necessary to identify and characterize each gene and mutation which may influence the VKA dose. In this task, the VKA research on pest management can be helpful. Indeed, management of rodent population has to deal with VKA resistances as well as in human medicine. Many mechanisms of resistances are common in humans and rodents. Moreover, with the large use of vitamin K antagonist rodenticides, the resistant phenotype is over-represented in some rodent populations. Consequently, some resistance mechanisms with a low prevalence in the human population have a higher prevalence in rodent population; thus, they can be more studied in rodents.

After a rapid presentation of the basis of vitamin K and VKA mechanisms, this chapter presents the different methods to assess VKA resistance mechanisms. Then, an assessment of the VKA-resistant pathways described in humans and in different rodent species is performed.

2. Basis of vitamin K metabolism

2.1. Vitamin K

The name "vitamin K" gathers a great number of molecules. All vitamin K are based on a naphthoquinone core and are sorted in three classes, numbered from 1 to 3. The substitution on the carbon 3 of the core determinates the class of the vitamin K. Vitamin K1 is composed of only one molecule, the phylloquinone, where the carbon 3 is substituted by a phytyl moiety. It was the first vitamin K described in 1935 by Dam [4], and chemically identified and synthesized by Doisy [5]. Vitamin K2 regroups the menaquinones. The substitute is a chain of prenyl, and the number of prenyls is indicated in the name. For example, the menaquinone 4 side chain is composed of 4 prenyl. Finally, vitamin K3 or menadione is only constituted by the naphthoquinone core (**Figure 1**).

Phylloquinone is synthesized by plants [6]. Menaquinones are synthesized from phylloquinone. The number of prenyls of the synthesized menaquinone depends on the bacteria, fungi, and animals which synthesize them. Mammals are only able to synthesize menaquinone 4 with

http://dx.doi.org/10.5772/64204

the help of the *UBIAD1* gene [7, 8]. Consequently, other menaquinone forms come mainly from fermented alimentation or gut microbial synthesis [9, 10].

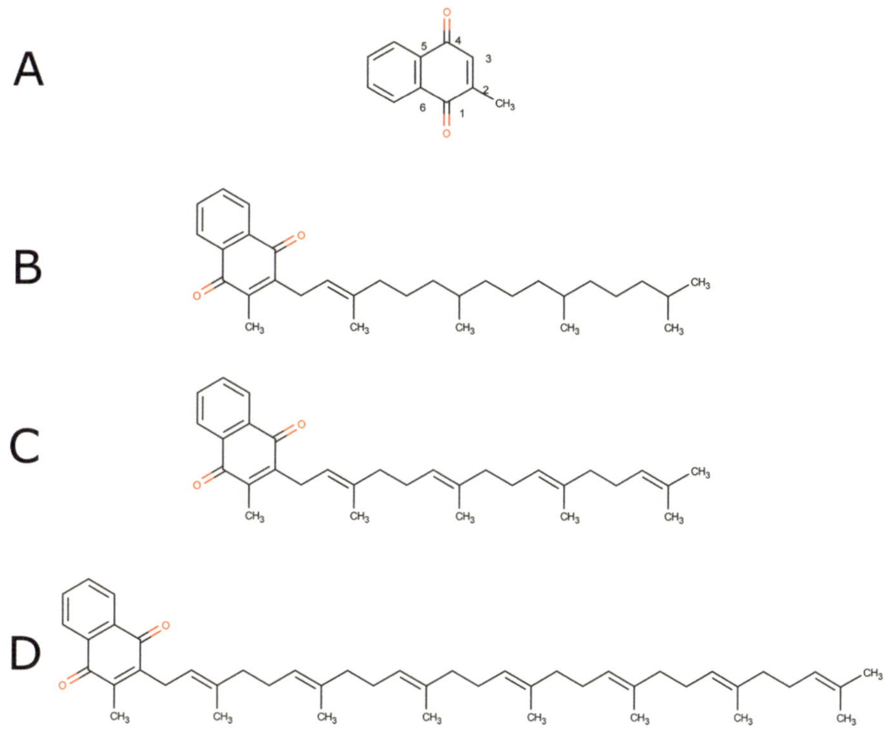

Figure 1. Examples of vitamin K: (A) menadione; (B) phylloquinone; (C) menaquinone 4; (D) menaquinone 7.

As many other fat-soluble vitamins, vitamin K's absorption increases with fatty intake [11]. The absorption of vitamin K occurs in the gut, nevertheless its mechanism has been unclear during many years [12]. Recently, a study suggested that the cholesterol transporter, the Niemann-Pick C1-like 1 protein, would be responsible for the vitamin K's absorption [13].

2.2. Vitamin K roles

The name of the vitamin K comes from the German word "koagulation." Indeed, when vitamin K was discovered, its deficiency involved bleeding [4]. Nevertheless, it is only in the 1970s that we began to understand the vitamin K's mechanism of action. Vitamin K is a cofactor of a post-transcriptional gamma-carboxylation which activates vitamin-K dependent proteins (VKDP) [14]. Four clotting factors of the coagulation cascade are the VKDPs, factors II, VII, IX, and X, which explain the bleeding issues observed in case of deficiency. Proteins C, S, and Z are also VKDPs involved in coagulation, but they have an antithrombotic effect. Nevertheless, the main effect of VKA is anticoagulation, even though the rapid decrease of these antithrombotic molecules can lead to a transient hypercoagulable state at the beginning or at the end of treatment with possible adverse events [15, 16].

The second great role of vitamin K is bone regulation with two VKDPs: osteocalcin and matrix GLA protein [17, 18]. This last protein is also involved in the protection against tissue calcification [19]. Vitamin K is involved in many other biological functions which are reviewed in Refs. [20, 21].

2.3. Vitamin K regeneration cycle

2.3.1. Vitamin K cycle

In spite of the low vitamin K level in food, vitamin K deficiency is rare [22]. Indeed, vitamin K is recycled by cells. The cycle is composed of two great steps: the use of vitamin K hydroquinone by the GGCX enzyme to activate VKDPs and the regeneration of the vitamin K hydroquinone from the epoxide form by VKORC1 (**Figure 2**).

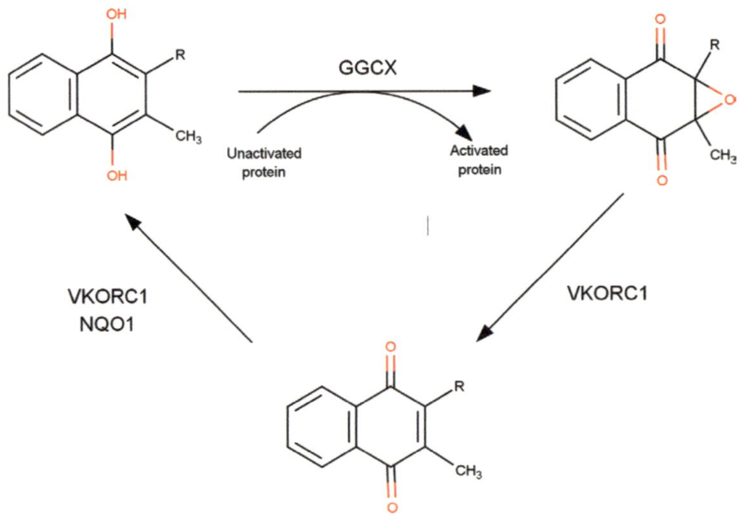

Figure 2. Vitamin K regeneration cycle.

In order to chelate calcium and to be active, the glutamate residues (Glu) of VKDPs have to be carboxylated to carboxyglutamic acid (Gla). This reaction is mediated by gamma-glutamyl carboxylase (GGCX). GGCX recognizes the VKDPs with the the help of their propeptide [23, 24]. Then, GGCX removes the gamma-hydrogen of Glu residues and adds CO_2; the oxidation of vitamin K hydroquinone (KH_2) to vitamin K epoxide ($K > 0$) provides the required energy [25]. This reaction is performed in the endoplasmic reticulum [26].

2.3.2. VKORC1 structure

The *VKORC1* gene was located in 1969 on the chromosome 1 of rat by discovering a link between the coat color heritage and the resistance to warfarin [27]. Then it was located on the chromosome 7 of mice in 1976 [28] and on the human chromosome 16 in 2002 [29]. The first characterization of the *VKORC1* activity was performed in 1974; nevertheless, at this time the responsible protein of this activity was unknown [30]. The identification of the *VKORC1* coding gene has only been performed in 2004 by two teams: one used short interference RNA functional screening [31] and the other used interspecies genetic linkage analysis [32]. Once identified and sequenced, the VKORC1's structure and function study begun.

A complete review of the current knowledge on the VKORC1 structure has been recently done [33]. VKORC1 is a membrane protein of the endoplasmic reticulum. The activity of VKORC1 seems to be due to CXXC patterns. VKORC1 presents two CXXC patterns, with cysteines positioned at Cys43, Cys51, Cys132, and Cys135 in human VKORC1. These cysteines are widely conserved through species, which might indicate that they have a key role in VKOR activity [34]. Cys132 and Cys135 are located in a transmembrane domain. They seem to be essential for the VKORC1 activity and might lead the nucleophilic attack supposed by a biochemical model of the VKOR reaction [34, 35]. Mutation of one of them to serine abolishes the enzymatic VKOR activity [36]. To reduce vitamin K, VKORC1 needs to be itself reduced by aphysiological partner. This partner and its mechanism of action are currently unknown. Schulman et al. proposed that the partner might reduce the loop cysteines (Cys43 and Cys51). Then the loop cysteines would transfer the reducing power to Cys132 and Cys135 of the active site [37]. However, other studies have reported that the mutation of one of these cysteines to serine has no consequence on the VKORC1 activity [38–40]. Moreover, the conformation of VKORC1 is still under debate between a topology with three transmembrane domains or four [41]. This last point is determining for the comprehension of the possible role of the loop cysteines. Indeed, they are either in the cytosol for the three transmembrane model or in the endoplasmic reticulum's lumen for the other model.

VKORC1 presents a strong homology between rodents and humans, allowing to compare the mutation between them. Mammals and bacterial VKORs are homologs, but their conformation and reaction seem different [42].

Mammals have another enzyme able to reduce the vitamin K epoxide, the VKORC1L1. It is mainly expressed in the extrahepatic tissues [43–45] and has a great similarity with VKORC1 [46]. Its inhibition by VKA is lower than its homolog [43]. Nevertheless, due to its low hepatic expression, its influence on the anticoagulant resistance is negligible. However, it might explain that the other vitamin K functions are not significantly impacted by VKA treatments.

2.4. Vitamin K antagonists

First VKA has been discovered in 1941 and then isolated in spoiled sweet clover by Hueber and Link [47]. Sweet clover (*Melilotus officinalis*) contains coumarin. In a poorly preserved silage or hay, this coumarin can be changed to dicoumarol by *Penicillium* species commonly present in soil [48, 49]. The dicoumarol contained in spoiled forage causes a hemorrhagic condition called sweet clover disease. Some years after this discovery, Coumadin, a synthetic VKA also called warfarin, was synthesized [50]. This last molecule is still the most commonly prescribed anticoagulant. Concerning rodents, many new VKA have been developed to reply to resistance emergence.

Three VKA families are used: the 4-hydroxycoumarin derivatives, the 4-hydroxy-thiocoumarin derivatives, and the indane-1,3-dione derivatives (**Figure 3**). All derivatives are used against rodents. Conversely, in human medicine, only the 4-hydroxycoumarin derivatives (for instance, warfarin) and the indane-1,3-dione derivatives (for instance, fluindione) are used. Moreover, in order to deal with rodent resistances, second generation of 4-hydroxycoumarin derivatives and of 4-hydroxy-thiocoumarin derivatives have been designed with complex radicals (**Figure 3C** and **D**).

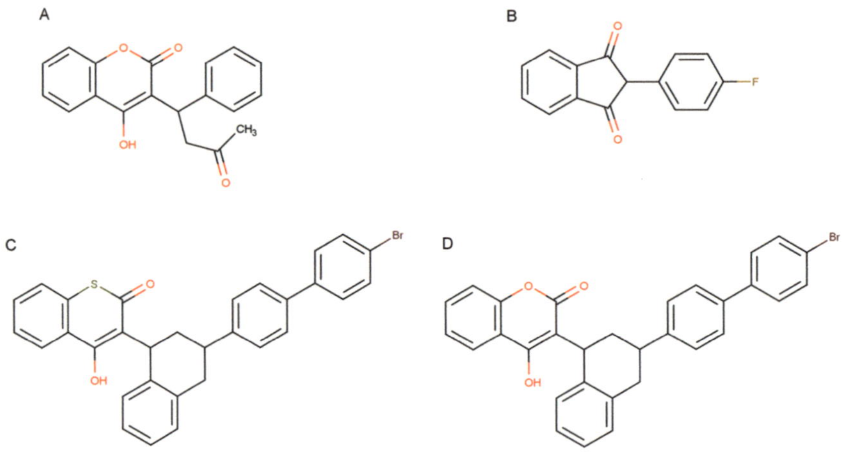

Figure 3. Examples of some VKA: (A) warfarin; (B) fluindione; (C) difethialone; (D) brodifacoum.

2.4.1. Mechanism of VKA action

Vitamin K antagonists stop the vitamin K recycling by performing noncompetitive inhibition of the VKORC1 enzyme [51, 52]. Nevertheless, the binding of VKA with VKORC1 enzyme is still a gray area. The reversibility of the binding is presently unknown [52–54], as well as the binding site. First, the binding site has been located at the level of the TYA motif (residues 138–140 in human VKORC1) close to the CXXC active site. Indeed, the mutation of the 139 tyrosine of this motif is associated with warfarin resistance in humans and rodents [55, 56], and by analogy the dicoumarol's binding site on NQO1 is also a TYA motif [57]. However, these mutations are moderately susceptible to second generation VKAs in rats [55, 58], which can suggest that other amino acids might be involved in this binding. Recently, Czogalla et al. have proposed a model involving three binding interfaces between warfarin and human VKORC1 [59].

2.4.2. VKA elimination pathway

The VKA treatments are established on the long term. Consequently, their elimination is a key factor which determines their liver concentration and finally their efficiency. The elimination pathway seems to depend on the molecule and on its enantiomeric form. Indeed, enantiomers of warfarin are eliminated differently. The (S)-enantiomer is metabolized exclusively by the hepatic cytochrome P450 isoform 2C9 (CYP2C9), while (R)-enantiomer is metabolized by isoforms CYP1A2, CYP2C19, CYP3A, and hepatic ketoreductase [60, 61]. Although the (R)-enantiomer has a longer half-life, it is less efficient, and the modulation of its elimination has no significant impact on the coagulation [62–64]. However, the activity of CYP2C9 is critical in the determination of the warfarin dose. Indeed, CYP2C9 activity is influenced by many drug interactions [65–68], and polymorphism of CYP2C9 can also modulate the sensitivity to warfarin.

3. Assess the resistances

Since the discovery of rats that are resistant to warfarin in 1960 by Boyle [69], the assessment and the study of resistance mechanisms have become a key issue for the rodent population management and in human medicine. Many methods have been developed to study these resistance mechanisms. Their purpose is to isolate the possible origins of the resistance in a standardized model and to evaluate if the induced resistance factor is of the same order as that one observed *in vivo*. The resistance factor is the factor by which the dose or concentration of VKA required for a susceptible population must be multiplied to achieve the same effect within a resistant population. We present below the main methods, and for each we pinpoint its advantages and limits.

3.1. *In vivo* animal studies

In vivo studies were commonly used in rodent VKA research in order to evaluate the efficiency of an anticoagulant or the consequences of *VKORC1* mutations. The first resistance case in rodents was assessed by Boyle. He fed suspected resistant with containing VKA food and control rats during 5 days. Then, the death rate between the two groups was compared [69]. This kind of survival challenge is efficient to qualify a resistance state and remains the gold standard to test commercial rodenticides. Nevertheless, these tests are long and have many shortcomings concerning animal welfare and the repeatability. Moreover, it is difficult with this test to compare two VKAs and to assess the dose–response law.

Later, new methods based on blood clotting test have been developed [70–72]. They were standardized by the Rodenticide Resistance Action Committee in order to obtain a discriminating dose for each VKA [73]. These doses of anticoagulants, called effective doses 50 (ED50), were determined to quantify the susceptibility of rats to anticoagulants. ED50 is the dose leading to 50% of animals tested with a fivefold increase of the international normalized ratio 24 h after the administration of anticoagulants. This technique is more precise and rapid. Nevertheless, this method gives few information on the mechanism of resistance.

The origins of resistances in wild strain can be multifactorial. For example, they can involve VKORC1-linked resistance and cytochrome-linked resistance. It is possible to refine *in vivo* methods by introgressing the studied wild mutation in laboratory stain. With this method, it is possible to isolate the resistant mutation in a susceptible genetic background [55].

If the animal *in vivo* studies are still the gold standard to the understanding of the complex effect of VKAs and of resistant mutations, they are expensive and laborious in the preparation and care of the strain and in the realization of experiments. Moreover, it may be interesting to study more precisely each mechanism by *in vitro* methods [74].

3.2. *In vitro* enzymatic study

The VKOR activity can be reproduced *in vitro*. These methods are based on the kinetics of vitamin K quinone production by an enzyme system from vitamin K > O. To perform this reaction, the substrate (vitamin K > O) is beforehand synthesized according to the method described by Tishler et al. [75]. The evaluated enzyme can come from animal tissues or heterologous expression culture (cell, bacteria, yeast, etc.). Finally, dithiothreitol (DTT) is commonly used to transfer the reduction power to the enzyme. The studied VKOR-specific activity and the Michaelis constant are calculated [76]. It is also possible to add VKA to study its inhibition efficiency. In this case, an inhibition constant can be obtained for each couple of enzymatic system and VKA. Methods to perform these experiments are described in Refs. [43, 58, 76].

This simple experiment pattern allows us to assess the efficiency of large origins of enzymatic system. As the VKOR proteins are located in the membrane of the endoplasmic reticulum, they are present in the microsomal fraction of tissues. The commonly used microsomal preparation methods are described in Ref. [76]. Microsomes are prepared from other cell components by differential centrifugation. Microsomal enzymatic activity evaluates the enzymatic efficiency of whole microsomal VKOR activity and not only of the VKORC1 enzyme activity. Indeed, Hammed et al. have pinpointed that a modeling with two enzymes (VKORC1L1 and VKORC1) is necessary to explain the inhibition of the testis microsomal activity by warfarin [43]. Moreover, as for *in vivo* experiment, the strains with interesting mutations have to be selected and preserved.

To isolate the activity of one enzyme or to perform enzymatic activity with human-like enzyme or mutated enzyme, it is possible to perform a heterologous expression in yeast (*Pichia pastoris*) of VKOR enzymes and then extract the yeast's microsomes. The method is described in Ref. [58]. Yeast has neither endogenous VKORC1 nor VKORC1L1. Thus, this method allows the study of the influence of VKORC1 and/or VKORC1L1 mutation on their respective specific activities and VKA resistance without interaction. The yeast model has been validated for some mutations as Y139F for which the resistance rate of rat's liver microsomes is the same as that of yeast microsomes. Moreover, it is also possible to test some hypothetic mutations. The yeast expression method is more focused on the enzyme activity than tissue microsomes and opens many experimental opportunities. However, the studied activity is still the microsome activity. With the previous methods, enzymes are in their microsomal environment. In order to study more precisely VKORC1-linked resistances, it would be interesting to purify VKORC1.

The purification of VKORC1 was for many years a big business [77, 78]. Indeed, this enzyme loses its activity during the solubilization. It was only in 2006 than Chu et al. have purified the recombinant human VKORC1 produced from a baculovirus in insect cells which was still active after purification [79]. In this experiment, microsomes were washed from non-VKORC1 proteins. The artificial membrane inclusion of VKORC1 after heterologous expression in *Escherichia coli*, its extraction, and its purification have recently been described [80]. Briefly, the *hVKORC1* gene has been expressed in *E. coli* BL21(DE3) in a KSI–hVKORC1–His_6 construct [81]. The ketosteroid isomerase (KSI) part promotes the expression of the protein in insoluble inclusion bodies. KSI part was linked with hVKORC1 by a formic acid cleavage site. Finally, the construct was hexahistidine-tagged. After the expression, proteins were preserved under denaturing conditions and purified with a HisTrap Ni-NTA column. Then the KSI part is removed with formic acid. The refolding of hVKORC1 was performed with pulsated renaturation and "artificial chaperone." Then the proteins were incorporated in a lipid layer to form a liposome. Jaeneke reported that the obtained hVKORC1 liposome had only 10% of the specific activity of the enzyme obtained with HEK293 cell [80]. These new purification methods are not currently used in the resistance study and need improvement. Nevertheless, they open the way for a better understanding of the VKORC1 topology and the influence of mutations on VKOR activity.

The enzymology studies are the basis of our current understanding of VKORC1 mutations and interaction with VKA. It is currently the technique with the best reproducibility and more reliability. Nevertheless, some issues are still pending with these methods. The major issue comes from the DTT which gives the reducing power to VKORC1 in experiments. DTT is a powerful reductor which might bypass some dysfunctional mechanisms of mutated enzyme by directly activating the active site [37]. Moreover, high concentration of DTT (>1 mM) add a background level. To limit it, Krettler et al. proposed the use of tris(3-hydroxypropyl)phosphine instead of DTT [82]. Nevertheless, there is not enough knowledge currently on this new methods and its VKORC1 interaction to change the method. Moreover, tris(3-hydroxypropyl)phosphine is less efficient in VKORC1 enzyme reduction than DTT at usual concentration.

Another issue might be that these methods study only the impact of VKA and resistant VKORC1 enzyme on the vitamin K regeneration cycle and not on the vitamin K-dependent protein gamma carboxylation. The required lipid environment and detergents are different for the activity between GGCX and VKORC1. Thus, it is currently difficult to study the interaction between both enzymes in an *in vitro* enzymatic assay [83]. These discrepancies imply that enzymology results have to be analyzed in view of the *in vivo* results.

3.3. *In vitro* cell study

In order to evaluate the complete reaction from vitamin K reduction to gamma-carboxylation and to solve some enzymatic study issues, the functional study of the vitamin K cycle in mammalian cells has been recently developed by Tie et al. [83], which was then adapted by other teams [84, 85]. In these studies, the production of a complete carboxylated protein by cell culture was assessed. The cells were HEK 293 cells transfected with the studied *VKORC1* gene and a VKDP. Then, cells were cultured in an environment containing vitamin K epoxide and the studied VKA. All methods have followed the gamma-carboxylation of factor IX gla domain by its monoclonal antibodies recognition [86] or by measuring its activity (only for complete factor IX). Three different vitamin K-dependent proteins have been used: the simple factor IX protein (FIX) [59, 84, 87]; the chimeric protein FactIXGLA, which was protein C with its gla domain replaced by the factor IX gla domain [40, 83]; the chimeric protein FIXgla-PRGP2, as previously the gla domain of the proline-rich gla protein was replaced by FIXgla domain [85]. Concerning the method using FIX [84, 87], the gamma-carboxylation was assessed by measuring the clotting activity of the concentrated culture medium mixed with factor IX-depleted plasma. For the FIXgla-PC method [40, 83], quantification is performed on the culture medium by an enzyme-linked immunosorbent assay (ELISA) with anti-FIXgla domain antibodies as coating antibodies. Although Jamil also used a chimeric protein transformed with a FIXgla domain for its quantification, in this case, it was the membrane protein, the proline-rich Gla protein 2, which was used. With this modification, carboxylated protein gla domains were presented at the surface of the cell, then recognized by monoclonal antibody conjugated to allophycocyanin and quantified by flow cytometer [85].

This new method is not standardized yet, and there is still a gray area in the interpretation of the obtained results. Indeed, some discrepancies exist between enzymatic assay and cell assay results [84, 88] and even between cell assay results [40, 59]. The origin of these discrepancies might be the interference of the cell's endogenous enzymes, in particular VKORC1L1, which is naturally more resistant than the wild VKORC1 enzyme [43]. In this way, standard cell assays have showed that all tested mutations were resistant [59, 84]. Tie et al. have dealt with this by knocking out endogenous *VKORC1* and *VKORC1L1* genes, using the transcription activator-like effector nuclease technology [40]. Thus, Tie et al. have confirmed the interaction of the endogenous enzyme in the cell assay, and they have showed that some mutations previously classed as resistant by Czogalla et al. [59] are in fact not resistant [40].

The second issue for the interpretation of cell assay is the lack of knowledge and control on it. This kind of assay is more complex than simple enzymatic activity; it involves many mechanisms that are currently uncontrolled or unknown: the level of the recombinant VKORC1 enzymes and the recombinant VKDP; the quantity and the efficiency of the physiological partner of VKOR enzymes, which are still unknown; the level of the endogenous GGCX protein; finally, the possible other mechanisms currently undescribed. All these elements determine if the studied enzymes are not bypassed and if the vitamin K reduction is the limiting reaction. These two conditions have to be fulfilled to validate completely the cell assay. However, some studies have pinpointed that the limiting reaction might be the VKORC1 enzyme reduction by its physiological partner and not the vitamin K reduction [89–91].

Although cell assays are recent and still have a gray area in the interpretation of their results, there is no doubt that they will become a key element of the study of VKA resistance mechanisms.

3.4. Pharmacogenomics study

The pharmacogenomics studies are the main source of *in vivo* information on the VKA resistance in humans. These studies assess the correlation between some genetic parameters and the warfarin dose, which allows to keep the patient's INR in the target zone. Among these parameters, the VKORC1 and the CYP2C9 polymorphisms are keys. But many other parameters, which might influence the VKA susceptibility, are unknown and cannot be evaluated by these studies. Pharmacogenomics studies assess the epidemiology of the mutations linked to resistance and can help in the determination of the treatment's starting dose by taking in account of patient's genome. But, their contribution to the study of the resistance pathway is limited to the confirmation or not of the results obtained with other methods.

4. Resistance pathways

4.1. VKOR-linked resistances

4.1.1. VKORC1 human genotypes

The pharmacogenomic studies and the reports of warfarin treatment failures have pinpointed two kinds of polymorphisms linked to VKORC1 which influence the warfarin dose requirements. The first is linked to the polymorphism in the noncoding region and the second is linked to missense mutations.

The polymorphism in the noncoding region is the origin of the majority of VKA dose variations [92–95]. Indeed, the noncoding region influences the transcription level of VKORC1 [94]. Nevertheless, these variations are minor, few milligrams of increase or decrease. So, it is not really resistance to VKA, but rather a slight modulation of VKA sensibility.

Conversely, the VKORC1 coding mutations are rare, and some involve a real resistance to VKA. They are characterized by a dose to stabilize the anticoagulation, which is higher than the high-dose threshold defined by Watzka: phenprocoumon 3.0 mg/day, acenocoumarol 3.5 mg/day, warfarin (W) 7.1 mg/day, and fluindione 19.8 mg/day, for mean age patients [56]. Please note that the definition of warfarin resistance is not well-defined. Currently, there are more than 27 mutations that have been described in patients with high requirements of VKA dose. They are summarized in **Table 1**.

Mutation	Number of patients	Molecule	Dose (mg /day)	Stable anticoagulation	Ref.	Confirmation of resistance by *in vitro* method†
A26P	1	W	20	No	[106]	Yes [88]
		F	100	No		
A26T	1	W	6	No	[56]	No [88]
L27V	1	W	7	Yes	[107]	No [88]
		F	60	No		
H28Q	1	P	10	yes	[56]	No [88]
V29L	2	W	14	?	[32, 56]	
		P	26	Yes		
A34P	1	W	27	Yes	[108]	
D36Y	31	W	16.1 [3–36]*	~	[56, 96, 105, 106, 109	No [88]
		F	45	No		

Mutation	Number of patients	Molecule	Dose (mg /day)	Stable anticoagulation	Ref.	Confirmation of resistance by *in vitro* method†
		A	7	No	–112]	
		P	7 [6.9–7.1]	Yes		
D36G	1	W	20	Yes	[56]	No [88]
A41S	1	W	16	?	[94]	No [88]
V45A	1	W	45	No	[32]	No [88]
S52L	1	P	9	No	[113]	Yes [40]
S52W	1	P	10	Yes	[56]	No [40]
V54L	2	W	21 [10–32]	~	[105, 106]	Yes [88]
		F	60	No		
		A	8	No		
S56F	1	P	15	No	[56]	No [88]
R58G	1	W	34	?	[32]	No [88]
W59R	3	A	9.3 [8–12]	No	[113, 114]	Yes [40]
		P	9	No		
W59C	1	P	11	No	[56]	No [88]
W59L	1	P	15	No	[56]	Yes [40]
V66M	15	W	31.5 [20–42]**	Yes	[56, 103, 105, 106, 108]	No [40]
		P	9.5 [9–10]	~		
V66G	1	P	8	Yes	[56]	No [40]
H68Y	1	–	–	–	[115]	Yes [88]
G71A	1	P	6	No	[56]	No [40]
N77S	1	P	9	No	[56]	Yes [40]
N77Y	1	W	25	Yes	[56]	No [40]
I123N	1	P	21	No	[56]	Yes [88]
L128R	16	W	44	No	[32, 105, 106, 116]	Yes [40]
		F	80	No		
		A	13	No		
		P	30	No		
Y139H	1	P	9	No	[56]	Yes [88]

Adapted and completed with permission from Ref. [88].
* A case report, which includes a 2-year-old girl, is not included [117].
** A report of two cases was not used due to its imprecision on the doses [118].
† Results of the Oldenburg's team are not reported [59, 84].
? no data are present on the stabilization of the anticoagulation in study.
~ only some patients have a stabilization of their anticoagulation.

Table 1. Genetic variations in the coding sequence of human VKORC1 in patients requiring high dose of a vitamin K antagonist.

Conversely, another mutation has been described by Rost in two Libyan families, the R98W mutation. Homozygous patients with this mutation have a combined deficiency of vitamin-K-dependent clotting factor type 2 which causes bleeding [32]. This deficiency can be treated by a daily dose of vitamin K. Rost et al. have shown in enzymatic assays that R98W-muted VKORC1, which was expressed in HEK cell, has a VKOR activity diminished of 90% [32].

Some mutations have a higher prevalence in some populations. Thus, the D36Y mutation is relatively well represented in some African populations [96]. The Ethiopian population and the Ashkenazi Jews population have a D36Y allele frequency of respectively 15% and 4% [97–99], while this mutation is absent in South African or in Chinese populations [100, 101]. Concerning the V66M mutation, it has been described in African and African-descent populations [102–104]. Finally, the L128R mutation has been described in different families [32, 105].

Nevertheless, the other reported mutations have been described only one time and sometimes on patient with unstabilized anticoagulation. These elements reduce the possibilities to determine a resistance factor for each. Moreover, the mutations have been often described as fortuitous events of pharmacogenomics studies [94]. Finally, the interactions with other mutations on cytochromes, GGCX, or noncoding part of *VKORC1* genes can also modulate the warfarin dose and enhance or reduce the resistance. Thus, the assessment of these mutations only from case report entails a lot of bias.

In order to deal with the described bias, the *in vitro* results can be useful. The *in vitro* results from enzymology [88] and cell assays [40] have been reported in **Table 1**. Nevertheless, all mutations do not seem to be associated with resistance in *in vitro* assays. Only Oldenburg have found that all the VKORC1 coding mutations were resistant with a cell method assay; his results are not reported in the table [59, 84]. This discrepancy between assays might be due to the *VKORC1L1* gene as afore-explained in the description of the cell assays. Moreover, enzymology assay pinpoints that some mutations drastically diminish the VKOR activity of the enzyme [88], whereas cell assays do not [40]. The study of the paralog mutations in rodents may help to understand the real impact of these mutations on the resistance.

4.1.2. VKORC1 rodent genotypes

Resistances have evolved differently in rodents according to their species. Indeed, the anticoagulant pressure is exerted differently on each. These differences depend on the behavior of the rodents, and more particularly the feeding behavior. Thus, some rodents feed preferentially on one food source (rat), while others feed on many sources (house mice). Thus, rats eat a lot of poisoned grains, whereas mice eat few poisoned baits and dilute them with other food sources.

Resistances have been largely described in house mice (*Mus musculus*) and in Norway rat (*Rattus norvegicus*). VKORC1-linked resistances are due to missense mutations. They have been detected whereupon rodenticide treatment fails. Due to the purpose of the VKA rodenticides, their doses used for management of rodents are important. Consequently, only huge resistances have been pinpointed and then isolated by introgressing the concerned genes in laboratory strains. Thus, the noncoding mutations, which are involved in the modulation of VKA dose in humans, have not been described in rodents.

Concerning the Norway rat, it has been the first target of the VKA rodenticides and the first to develop resistances [69]. The first description occurred in Scotland, and rapidly the resistance spread all over Great Britain [119, 120]. Denmark has been the second country with warfarin-resistant rats [121]. Entrapments have pinpointed that 24.2% of Denmark's rats were resistant in the 1960s [122]. Since then, resistances have been brought to light from all around the world [123, 124].

Currently, 25 mutations have been described in Norway rats [125]. Nevertheless, only few mutations are widely present and linked with important resistances. The five main mutations in Europe are L120Q, L128Q, Y139C, Y139F, and Y139S [126]. These mutations have different frequencies depending on the geographical areas. Thus, Y139C is the main mutation in Germany and Denmark [126, 127], and Y139F in France [128]. Concerning Great Britain, important discrepancies on the frequencies of mutations have been pinpointed between counties [126, 129, 130]. The frequencies of rat mutations are disproportionate comparatively to human coding mutation frequency. Thus, Y139F mutation is detected in 21% of the French rats [128], but less than 1% of the world human population carries one coding mutation. Moreover, in some areas, the prevalence of the resistant rats is of 100% [131].

Concerning the house mice, their mutations have been described in 1961 in many countries [132]. Currently, more than 10 *VKORC1* mutations have been described [133]. Moreover, 80% of the trapped mice carried at least one *VKORC1* mutation in a study in Germany, Switzerland, and Azores [133]. Finally, some population of house mice have multiple mutations, Arg12Trp/Ala26Ser/Ala48Thr/Arg61Leu, which involve VKA resistance [133]. This mutation may come from an interspecific hybridization with *Mus spretus*. But, only little information is available on *Mus spretus*'s resistance to VKA [133].

4.1.3. Overall approach of human and rodent mutations

The presence of *VKORC1* mutations in humans with very low frequency (<1%) and the fast emergence of resistance in rodents indicate that the mutations were present in rodents well before the use of VKA as rodenticide. The large use of these molecules has selected the resistant mutations of *VKORC1* and increased their prevalence in rodent populations. Moreover, the use of excessive dose of VKA has selected the mutations leading to the most severe resistance, especially in *Rattus norvegicus* populations. Indeed, in Europe, while more than 20 mutations were published, only three mutations seem now widely spread. As the roof rat population is less exposed to VKA than brown rats, the prevalence of their *VKORC1* mutations might be close to human prevalence. The roof rat resistance linked to *VKORC1* mutation has not been widely explored. Recently, Goulois has characterized the Y25F mutation in roof rats [134].

Five amino acid positions of the VKORC1 enzyme carry a described mutation in both humans and rodents. They are the positions A26, R58, W59, L128, and Y139. Nevertheless, only the mutations A26T, R58G, and W59R are identical. These three mutations are not common in humans, and the reported cases did not have a stable anticoagulation. The A26T mutation does not seem to enhance the resistance in the rat [125]. These results were obtained with rat *VKORC1* cell expression, and they agree with the results obtained with human *VKORC1* [88]. Moreover, the frequency of this mutation is low in rats which might suggest that the resistance linked to this mutation is insufficient to be selected by the VKA rodenticide pressure. Concerning the W59R mutation, it diminishes considerably the VKOR activity of the enzyme in rats conversely to in humans [40, 125]. Finally, R58G mutation is described both in humans and mice. This mutation does not seem to involve resistance in mice, and as the W59R mutation in rat, it diminishes the VKOR activity [125]. Thus, the results obtained with VKORC1 enzyme of rodents are in accordance with the *in vitro* results with human *VKORC1* gene or VKORC1 enzyme.

The mutations at positions L128 and Y139 are the major mutations of the Norway rat. Moreover, the studies on the Y139F mutations have shown that the resistance factor of this mutation is conserved between *in vivo* and *in vitro* assays [55, 58]. In rats, these mutations involve resistance factors against warfarin, which are of 8 for the L128Q mutation and greater than 200 for the Y139 mutations [58]. Moreover, in rats, L128Q does not seem to diminish the VKOR activity while Y139F does it. Conversely, in humans, the L128R mutation conducts to a reduction of more than 90% of the VKOR activity in enzymatic assay, with the VKORC1 enzyme produced in yeasts or HEK cells [32, 88]. But, this mutation does not modify the level of gamma-carboxylation in cell assay [40, 84]. Possible origins of these discrepancies are argued in Section 3.3. Consequently, it is currently difficult to conclude on the possible resistance linked with the L128R mutation in humans.

As aforementioned, some mutations decrease the efficiency of the VKOR activity. Matagrin has studied the origins of this loss of efficiency for the Y139 mutation [135]. He showed that Y139 mutations involve a diminution of the VKOR activity and the creation of inactive vitamin K metabolites (3-OH vitamin K) which are eliminated. This induces an increase of the food requirements of vitamin K in rodents carrying these mutations [136, 137]. In humans, the influence of coding mutations on nutritional requirement of vitamin K has not been well studied [22]. However, by analogy with rodent mutations, human mutations might be involved in cardiovascular diseases without VKA treatment [138]. Thus, the rodents carrying these mutations might be use to model and to better understand the possible consequences of these mutations on the human health.

4.2. Cytochrome-linked resistances

Cytochromes are essential elements in the elimination of xenobiotics. Thus, it would be expected that their polymorphism might result in an origin of resistances. But in human medicine, the cytochrome polymorphism is associated with an increase in the patient's VKA sensibility [93, 97]. Moreover, the polymorphism of CYP2C9 is a key element in the prediction of the VKA treatment dose [97]. Thus, no VKA resistance linked to cytochrome has been described in human medicine.

In rodents, expression profiles of cytochromes are different between sensitive and resistant rats carrying a Y139C mutation on VKORC1 [139]. Nevertheless, it is difficult to identify the part of the resistance due to VKORC1 mutation and the one due to the expression profiles of cytochromes. Nevertheless, one example of warfarin resistance linked to cytochrome has been described without association with VKORC1 mutation in roof rats from Tokyo [140, 141]. This rat population overexpresses the cytochrome 3A2. Thus, the concentration of blood warfarin 1 h after the warfarin administration is eightfold lower in resistant rats. However, it is currently the only reported case of cytochrome-linked resistance.

5. Conclusion

The assessment and the comprehension of the resistance mechanisms are essential in the safety and the efficiency of VKA treatments and in the rodent population management. However, the complexity of the mechanisms and the interactions between them prevent the use of only one studying method. The understanding of the VKA actions and their interaction with individual variability can only be achieved by a multiscale approach which combines humans, rodents, and *in vitro* and *in vivo* knowledge.

Author details

Sébastien Lefebvre, Etienne Benoit and Virginie Lattard*

*Address all correspondence to: virginie.lattard@vetagro-sup.fr

USC 1233 INRA-Vetagro Sup, Veterinary School of Lyon, Marcy l'Etoile, France

References

[1] Fareed J. Antithrombotic therapy in 2014: Making headway in anticoagulant and antiplatelet therapy. Nat Rev Cardiol. 2015;12(2):70–1.

[2] Kuruvilla M, Gurk-Turner C. A review of warfarin dosing and monitoring. Proc Bayl Univ Med Cent. 2001;14(3):305–6.

[3] Wysowski DK, Nourjah P, Swartz L. Bleeding complications with warfarin use: A prevalent adverse effect resulting in regulatory action. Arch Intern Med. 2007;167(13): 1414–9.

[4] Dam H. The antihaemorrhagic vitamin of the chick. Biochem J. 1935;29(6):1273–85.

[5] MacCorquodale DW, Binkley SB, Thayer SA, Doisy EA. On the constitution of vitamin K1. J Am Chem Soc. 1939;61(7):1928–9.

[6] Widhalm JR, Ducluzeau A-L, Buller NE, Elowsky CG, Olsen LJ, Basset GJC. Phylloquinone (vitamin K1) biosynthesis in plants: Two peroxisomal thioesterases of lactobacillales origin hydrolyze 1,4-dihydroxy-2-naphthoyl-coa. Plant J. 2012;71(2):205–15.

[7] Okano T, Shimomura Y, Yamane M, Suhara Y, Kamao M, Sugiura M, et al. Conversion of Phylloquinone (Vitamin K1) into Menaquinone-4 (Vitamin K2) in Mice two possible routes for menaquinone-4 accumulation in cerebra of mice. J Biol Chem. 2008;283(17): 11270–9.

[8] Nakagawa K, Hirota Y, Sawada N, Yuge N, Watanabe M, Uchino Y, et al. Identification of UBIAD1 as a novel human menaquinone-4 biosynthetic enzyme. Nature. 2010;468(7320):117–21.

[9] Conly JM, Stein K. The production of menaquinones (vitamin K2) by intestinal bacteria and their role in maintaining coagulation homeostasis. Prog Food Nutr Sci. 1992;16(4): 307–43.

[10] LeBlanc JG, Milani C, de Giori GS, Sesma F, van Sinderen D, Ventura M. Bacteria as vitamin suppliers to their host: A gut microbiota perspective. Curr Opin Biotechnol. 2013;24(2):160–8.

[11] Gijsbers BL, Jie KS, Vermeer C. Effect of food composition on vitamin K absorption in human volunteers. Br J Nutr. 1996;76(2):223–9.

[12] Reboul E, Borel P. Proteins involved in uptake, intracellular transport and basolateral secretion of fat-soluble vitamins and carotenoids by mammalian enterocytes. Prog Lipid Res. 2011;50(4):388–402.

[13] Takada T, Yamanashi Y, Konishi K, Yamamoto T, Toyoda Y, Masuo Y, et al. NPC1L1 is a key regulator of intestinal vitamin K absorption and a modulator of warfarin therapy. Sci Transl Med. 2015;7(275):275ra23.

[14] Stenflo J, Fernlund P, Egan W, Roepstorff P. Vitamin K dependent modifications of glutamic acid residues in prothrombin. Proc Natl Acad Sci U S A. 1974;71(7):2730–3.

[15] Grip L, Blombäck M, Schulman S. Hypercoagulable state and thromboembolism following warfarin withdrawal in post-myocardial-infarction patients. Eur Heart J. 1991;12(11):1225–33.

[16] Azoulay L, Dell'Aniello S, Simon TA, Renoux C, Suissa S. Initiation of warfarin in patients with atrial fibrillation: Early effects on ischaemic strokes. Eur Heart J. 2014;35(28):1881–7.

[17] Vermeer C, Jie K-SG, Knapen MHJ. Role of vitamin K in bone metabolism. Annu Rev Nutr. 1995;15(1):1–21.

[18] Ferron M, Lacombe J, Germain A, Oury F, Karsenty G. GGCX and VKORC1 inhibit osteocalcin endocrine functions. J Cell Biol. 2015;208(6):761–76.

[19] Luo G, Ducy P, McKee MD, Pinero GJ, Loyer E, Behringer RR, et al. Spontaneous calcification of arteries and cartilage in mice lacking matrix GLA protein. Nature. 1997;386(6620):78–81.

[20] Ferland G. Vitamin K and the nervous system: An overview of its actions. Adv Nutr. 2012;3(2):204–12.

[21] Booth SL. Roles for vitamin K beyond coagulation. Annu Rev Nutr. 2009;29(1):89–110.

[22] Shearer MJ, Fu X, Booth SL. Vitamin K nutrition, metabolism, and requirements: Current concepts and future research. Adv Nutr Int Rev J. 2012;3(2):182–95.

[23] Pan LC, Price PA. The propeptide of rat bone gamma-carboxyglutamic acid protein shares homology with other vitamin K-dependent protein precursors. Proc Natl Acad Sci U S A. 1985;82(18):6109–13.

[24] Stanley TB, Jin DY, Lin PJ, Stafford DW. The propeptides of the vitamin K-dependent proteins possess different affinities for the vitamin K-dependent carboxylase. J Biol Chem. 1999;274(24):16940–4.

[25] Friedman PA, Shia MA, Gallop PM, Griep AE. Vitamin K-dependent gamma-carbon-hydrogen bond cleavage and nonmandatory concurrent carboxylation of peptide-bound glutamic acid residues. Proc Natl Acad Sci U S A. 1979;76(7):3126–9.

[26] Van Horn WD. Structural and functional insights into human vitamin K epoxide reductase and vitamin K epoxide reductase-like1. Crit Rev Biochem Mol Biol. 2013;48(4):357–72.

[27] Greaves JH, Ayres P. Linkages between genes for coat colour and resistance to warfarin in Rattus norvegicus. Nature. 1969;224(5216):284–5.

[28] Wallace ME, MacSwiney FJ. A major gene controlling warfarin-resistance in the house mouse. J Hyg (Lond). 1976;76(2):173–81.

[29] Fregin A, Rost S, Wolz W, Krebsova A, Muller CR, Oldenburg J. Homozygosity mapping of a second gene locus for hereditary combined deficiency of vitamin K–dependent clotting factors to the centromeric region of chromosome 16. Blood. 2002;100(9):3229–32.

[30] Zimmermann A, Matschiner JT. Biochemical basis of hereditary resistance to warfarin in the rat. Biochem Pharmacol. 1974;23(6):1033–40.

[31] Li T, Chang C-Y, Jin D-Y, Lin P-J, Khvorova A, Stafford DW. Identification of the gene for vitamin K epoxide reductase. Nature. 2004;427(6974):541–4.

[32] Rost S, Fregin A, Ivaskevicius V, Conzelmann E, Hörtnagel K, Pelz H-J, et al. Mutations in VKORC1 cause warfarin resistance and multiple coagulation factor deficiency type 2. Nature. 2004;427(6974):537–41.

[33] Tie J-K, Stafford DW. Structural and functional insights into enzymes of the vitamin K cycle. J Thromb Haemost. 2016;14(2):236–47.

[34] Goodstadt L, Ponting CP. Vitamin K epoxide reductase: Homology, active site and catalytic mechanism. Trends Biochem Sci. 2004;29(6):289–92.

[35] Silverman RB. Chemical model studies for the mechanism of vitamin K epoxide reductase. J Am Chem Soc. 1981;103(19):5939–41.

[36] Wajih N, Sane DC, Hutson SM, Wallin R. Engineering of a recombinant vitamin K-dependent γ-carboxylation system with enhanced γ-carboxyglutamic acid forming capacity evidence for a functional cxxc redox center in the system. J Biol Chem. 2005;280(11):10540–7.

[37] Schulman S, Wang B, Li W, Rapoport TA. Vitamin K epoxide reductase prefers ER membrane-anchored thioredoxin-like redox partners. Proc Natl Acad Sci U S A. 2010;107(34):15027–32.

[38] Jin D-Y, Tie J-K, Stafford DW. The conversion of vitamin K epoxide to vitamin K quinone and vitamin K quinone to vitamin K hydroquinone uses the same active site cysteines. Biochemistry (Mosc). 2007;46(24):7279–83.

[39] Rost S, Fregin A, Hünerberg M, Bevans CG, Müller CR, Oldenburg J. Site-directed mutagenesis of coumarin-type anticoagulant-sensitive VKORC1: Evidence that highly conserved amino acids define structural requirements for enzymatic activity and inhibition by warfarin. Thromb Haemost. 2005;94(4):780–6.

[40] Tie J-K, Jin D-Y, Tie K, Stafford DW. Evaluation of warfarin resistance using TALENs-mediated vitamin K epoxide reductase knockout HEK293 cells. J Thromb Haemost JTH. 2013;11(8):1556–64.

[41] Czogalla KJ, Watzka M, Oldenburg J. Structural modeling insights into human VKORC1 phenotypes. Nutrients. 2015;7(8):6837–51.

[42] Tie J-K, Jin D-Y, Stafford DW. Human vitamin K epoxide reductase and its bacterial homologue have different membrane topologies and reaction mechanisms. J Biol Chem. 2012;287(41):33945–55.

[43] Hammed A, Matagrin B, Spohn G, Prouillac C, Benoit E, Lattard V. VKORC1L1, an enzyme rescuing the vitamin K 2,3-epoxide reductase activity in some extrahepatic tissues during anticoagulation therapy. J Biol Chem. 2013;288(40):28733–42.

[44] Melé M, Ferreira PG, Reverter F, DeLuca DS, Monlong J, Sammeth M, et al. The human transcriptome across tissues and individuals. Science. 2015;348(6235):660–5.

[45] Caspers M, Czogalla KJ, Liphardt K, Müller J, Westhofen P, Watzka M, et al. Two enzymes catalyze vitamin K 2,3-epoxide reductase activity in mouse: VKORC1 is highly expressed in exocrine tissues while VKORC1L1 is highly expressed in brain. Thromb Res. 2015;135(5):977–83.

[46] Oldenburg J, Watzka M, Bevans CG. VKORC1 and VKORC1L1: Why do vertebrates have two vitamin K 2,3-epoxide reductases? Nutrients. 2015;7(8):6250–80.

[47] Huebner CF, Link KP. Studies on the hemorrhagic sweet clover disease VI. The synthesis of the δ-diketone derived from the hemorrhagic agent through alkaline degradation. J Biol Chem. 1941;138(2):529–34.

[48] Bellis DM. Metabolism of coumarin and related compounds in cultures of penicillium species. Nature. 1958;182:806–7.

[49] Goplen BP. Sweetclover production and agronomy. Can Vet J. 1980;21(5):149–51.

[50] Miyoshi I, Paul LK, Stahmann MA. 3-substituted 4-hydroxycoumarin and process of making it [Internet]. US2427578 A, 1947 [cité 27 mars 2015]. Disponible sur: http://www.google.fr/patents/US2427578

[51] Lasseur R, Longin-Sauvageon C, Videmann B, Billeret M, Berny P, Benoit E. Warfarin resistance in a French strain of rats. J Biochem Mol Toxicol. 2006;19(6): 379–85.

[52] Lorusso DJ, Suttie JW. Warfarin binding to microsomes isolated from normal and warfarin-resistant rat liver. Mol Pharmacol. 1972;8(2):197–203.

[53] Bevans CG, Krettler C, Reinhart C, Tran H, Koßmann K, Watzka M, et al. Determination of the warfarin inhibition constant Ki for vitamin K 2,3-epoxide reductase complex subunit-1 (VKORC1) using an *in vitro* DTT-driven assay. Biochim Biophys Acta BBA – Gen Subj. 2013;1830(8):4202–10.

[54] Thijssen HHW. Warfarin resistance: Vitamin K epoxide reductase of scottish resistance genes is not irreversibly blocked by warfarin. Biochem Pharmacol. 1987;36(17):2753–7.

[55] Grandemange A, Kohn MH, Lasseur R, Longin-Sauvageon C, Berny P, Benoit E. Consequences of the Y139F VKORC1 mutation on resistance to AVKs: In-vivo investigation in a 7th generation of congenic Y139F strain of rats. Pharmacogenet Genomics. 2009;19(10):742–50.

[56] Watzka M, Geisen C, Bevans CG, Sittinger K, Spohn G, Rost S, et al. Thirteen novel VKORC1 mutations associated with oral anticoagulant resistance: Insights into improved patient diagnosis and treatment. J Thromb Haemost. 2011;9(1): 109–18.

[57] Asher G, Dym O, Tsvetkov P, Adler J, Shaul Y. The crystal structure of NAD(P)H quinone oxidoreductase 1 in complex with its potent inhibitor dicoumarol. Biochemistry (Mosc). 2006;45(20):6372–8.

[58] Hodroge A, Longin-Sauvageon C, Fourel I, Benoit E, Lattard V. Biochemical characterization of spontaneous mutants of rat VKORC1 involved in the resistance to antivitamin K anticoagulants. Arch Biochem Biophys. 2011;515(1–2):14–20.

[59] Czogalla KJ, Biswas A, Wendeln A-C, Westhofen P, Müller CR, Watzka M, et al. Human VKORC1 mutations cause variable degrees of 4-hydroxycoumarin resistance and affect putative warfarin binding interfaces. Blood. 2013;122(15):2743–50.

[60] Kaminsky LS, Zhang Z-Y. Human P450 metabolism of warfarin. Pharmacol Ther. 1997;73(1):67–74.

[61] Rettie AE, Korzekwa KR, Kunze KL, Lawrence RF, Eddy AC, Aoyama T, et al. Hydroxylation of warfarin by human cDNA-expressed cytochrome P-450: A role for P-4502C9 in the etiology of (S)-warfarin-drug interactions. Chem Res Toxicol. 1992;5(1): 54–9.

[62] Breckenridge A, Orme M, Wesseling H, Lewis RJ, Gibbons R. Pharmacokinetics and pharmacodynamics of the enantiomers of warfarin in man. Clin Pharmacol Ther. 1974;15(4):424–30.

[63] O'Reilly RA. Studies on the optical enantiomorphs of warfarin in man. Clin Pharmacol Ther. 1974;16(2):348–54.

[64] Takahashi DH, Echizen H. Pharmacogenetics of warfarin elimination and its clinical implications. Clin Pharmacokinet. 2012;40(8):587–603.

[65] Black DJ, Kunze KL, Wienkers LC, Gidal BE, Seaton TL, McDonnell ND, et al. Warfarin-fluconazole. II. A metabolically based drug interaction: *In vivo* studies. Drug Metab Dispos. 1996;24(4):422–8.

[66] Kunze KL, Trager WF. Warfarin-fluconazole. III. A rational approach to management of a metabolically based drug interaction. Drug Metab Dispos. 1996;24(4):429–35.

[67] Wells PS, Holbrook AM, Crowther NR, Hirsh J. Interactions of warfarin with drugs and food. Ann Intern Med. 1994;121(9):676–83.

[68] Takahashi H, Kashima T, Kimura S, Murata N, Takaba T, Iwade K, et al. Pharmacokinetic interaction between warfarin and a uricosuric agent, bucolome: Application of *in vitro* approaches to predicting *in vivo* reduction of (s)-warfarin clearance. Drug Metab Dispos. 1999;27(10):1179–86.

[69] Boyle CM. Case of apparent resistance of rattus norvegicus berkenhout to anticoagulant poisons. Nature. 1960;188(4749):517–517.

[70] Gill JE, Kerins GM, Langton SD, MacNicoll AD. Blood-clotting response test for bromadiolone resistance in norway rats. J Wildl Manag. 1994;58(3):454–61.

[71] Macnicoll AD, Gill JE. Revised methodology for a blood-clotting response test for identification of warfarin-resistant Norway rats (Rattus norvegicus). EPPO Bull. 1993;23(4):701–7.

[72] Gill JE, Kerins GM, Langton SD, Macnicoll AD. The development of a blood clotting response test for discriminating between difenacoum-resistant and susceptible

Norway rats (Rattus norvegicus, berk.). Comp Biochem Physiol Part C Comp Pharmacol. 1993;104(1):29–36.

[73] Prescott CV. A Reappraisal of Blood Clotting Response Tests for Anticoagulant Resistance and a proposal for a standardised BCR Test Methodology. Brussel: CropLife international; 2003. 21 p. (Rodenticide Resistance Action Committee).

[74] Aithal GP, Day CP, Kesteven PJ, Daly AK. Association of polymorphisms in the cytochrome P450 CYP2C9 with warfarin dose requirement and risk of bleeding complications. The Lancet. 1999;353(9154):717–9.

[75] Tishler M, Fieser LF, Wendler NL. Hydro, Oxido and other derivatives of vitamin K1 and related compounds. J Am Chem Soc. 1940;62(10):2866–71.

[76] MacNicoll AD, Nadian AK, Townsend MG. Inhibition by warfarin of liver microsomal vitamin K-reductase in warfarin-resistant and susceptible rats. Biochem Pharmacol. 1984;33(8):1331–6.

[77] Begent LA, Hill AP, Steventon GB, Hutt AJ, Pallister CJ, Cowell DC. Characterization and purification of the vitamin K1 2,3 epoxide reductase system from rat liver. J Pharm Pharmacol. 2001;53(4):481–6.

[78] Guenthner TM, Cai D, Wallin R. Co-purification of microsomal epoxide hydrolase with the warfarin-sensitive vitamin K1 oxide reductase of the vitamin K cycle. Biochem Pharmacol. 1998;55(2):169–75.

[79] Chu P-H, Huang T-Y, Williams J, Stafford DW. Purified vitamin K epoxide reductase alone is sufficient for conversion of vitamin K epoxide to vitamin K and vitamin K to vitamin KH2. Proc Natl Acad Sci U S A. 2006;103(51):19308–13.

[80] Jaenecke F, Friedrich-Epler B, Parthier C, Stubbs MT. Membrane composition influences the activity of *in vitro* refolded human vitamin K epoxide reductase. Biochemistry (Mosc). 2015;54(42):6454–61.

[81] Banères J-L, Mesnier D, Martin A, Joubert L, Dumuis A, Bockaert J. Molecular characterization of a purified 5-ht4 receptor a structural basis for drug efficacy. J Biol Chem. 2005;280(21):20253–60.

[82] Krettler C, Bevans CG, Reinhart C, Watzka M, Oldenburg J. Tris(3-hydroxypropyl)phosphine is superior to dithiothreitol for *in vitro* assessment of vitamin K 2,3-epoxide reductase activity. Anal Biochem. 2015;474:89–94.

[83] Tie J-K, Jin D-Y, Straight DL, Stafford DW. Functional study of the vitamin K cycle in mammalian cells. Blood. 2011;117(10):2967–74.

[84] Fregin A, Czogalla KJ, Gansler J, Rost S, Taverna M, Watzka M, et al. A new cell culture-based assay quantifies vitamin K 2,3-epoxide reductase complex subunit 1 function and reveals warfarin resistance phenotypes not shown by the dithiothreitol-driven VKOR assay. J Thromb Haemost. 2013;11(5):872–80.

[85] Haque JA, McDonald MG, Kulman JD, Rettie AE. A cellular system for quantitation of vitamin K cycle activity: Structure-activity effects on vitamin K antagonism by warfarin metabolites. Blood. 2014;123(4):582–9.

[86] Aktimur A, Gabriel MA, Gailani D, Toomey JR. The factor IX γ-carboxyglutamic acid (gla) domain is involved in interactions between factor IX and factor XIa. J Biol Chem. 2003;278(10):7981–7.

[87] Müller E, Keller A, Fregin A, Müller CR, Rost S. Confirmation of warfarin resistance of naturally occurring VKORC1 variants by coexpression with coagulation factor IX and in silico protein modelling. BMC Genet. 2014;15:17.

[88] Hodroge A, Matagrin B, Moreau C, Fourel I, Hammed A, Benoit E, et al. VKORC1 mutations detected in patients resistant to vitamin K antagonists are not all associated with a resistant VKOR activity. J Thromb Haemost. 2012;10(12):2535–43.

[89] Sun Y-M, Jin D-Y, Camire RM, Stafford DW. Vitamin K epoxide reductase significantly improves carboxylation in a cell line overexpressing factor X. Blood. 2005;106(12):3811–5.

[90] Wajih N, Hutson SM, Owen J, Wallin R. Increased production of functional recombinant human clotting factor IX by baby hamster kidney cells engineered to overexpress VKORC1, the vitamin K 2,3-epoxide-reducing enzyme of the vitamin K cycle. J Biol Chem. 2005;280(36):31603–7.

[91] Hallgren KW, Qian W, Yakubenko AV, Runge KW, Berkner KL. r-VKORC1 expression in factor IX BHK cells increases the extent of factor IX carboxylation but is limited by saturation of another carboxylation component or by a shift in the rate-limiting step. Biochemistry (Mosc). 2006;45(17):5587–98.

[92] Gaio V, Picanço I, Nunes B, Fernandes A, Mendonça F, Horta Correia F, et al. Pharmacogenetic profile of a South Portuguese population: Results from the pilot study of the European Health Examination Survey in Portugal. Public Health Genomics. 2015;18(3):139–50.

[93] Giri AK, Khan NM, Grover S, Kaur I, Basu A, Tandon N, et al. Genetic epidemiology of pharmacogenetic variations in CYP2C9, CYP4F2 and VKORC1 genes associated with warfarin dosage in the Indian population. Pharmacogenomics. 2014;15(10):1337–54.

[94] Rieder MJ, Reiner AP, Gage BF, Nickerson DA, Eby CS, McLeod HL, et al. Effect of VKORC1 haplotypes on transcriptional regulation and warfarin dose. N Engl J Med. 2005;352(22):2285–93.

[95] Limdi NA, Beasley TM, Crowley MR, Goldstein JA, Rieder MJ, Flockhart DA, et al. VKORC1 polymorphisms, haplotypes and haplotype groups on warfarin dose among African–Americans and European–Americans. Pharmacogenomics. 2008;9(10):1445–58.

[96] Shahin MHA, Cavallari LH, Perera MA, Khalifa SI, Misher A, Langaee T, et al. VKORC1 Asp36Tyr geographic distribution and its impact on warfarin dose requirements in Egyptians. Thromb Haemost. 2013;109(6):1045–50.

[97] Scott SA, Edelmann L, Kornreich R, Desnick RJ. Warfarin pharmacogenetics: CYP2C9 and VKORC1 genotypes predict different sensitivity and resistance frequencies in the ashkenazi and sephardi jewish populations. Am J Hum Genet. 2008;82(2):495–500.

[98] Aklillu E, Leong C, Loebstein R, Halkin H, Gak E. VKORC1 Asp36Tyr warfarin resistance marker is common in Ethiopian individuals. Blood. 2008;111(7):3903–4.

[99] Sominsky S, Korostishevsky M, Kurnik D, Aklillu E, Cohen Y, Ken-Dror G, et al. The VKORC1 Asp36Tyr variant and VKORC1 haplotype diversity in Ashkenazi and Ethiopian populations. J Appl Genet. 2014;55(2):163–71.

[100] Mitchell C, Gregersen N, Krause A. Novel CYP2C9 and VKORC1 gene variants associated with warfarin dosage variability in the South African black population. Pharmacogenomics. 2011;12(7):953–63.

[101] Cen H-J, Zeng W-T, Leng X-Y, Huang M, Chen X, Li J-L, et al. CYP4F2 rs2108622: A minor significant genetic factor of warfarin dose in Han Chinese patients with mechanical heart valve replacement. Br J Clin Pharmacol. 2010;70(2):234–40.

[102] Suarez-Kurtz G, Botton MR. Pharmacogenomics of warfarin in populations of African descent. Br J Clin Pharmacol. 2013;75(2):334–46.

[103] Harrington DJ, Underwood S, Morse C, Shearer MJ, Tuddenham EGD, Mumford AD. Pharmacodynamic resistance to warfarin associated with a Val66Met substitution in vitamin K epoxide reductase complex subunit 1. Thromb Haemost. 2005;93(1):23–6.

[104] Scott SA, Jaremko M, Lubitz SA, Kornreich R, Halperin JL, Desnick RJ. CYP2C9*8 is prevalent among African–Americans: Implications for pharmacogenetic dosing. Pharmacogenomics. 2009;10(8):1243–55.

[105] Harrington DJ, Gorska R, Wheeler R, Davidson S, Murden S, Morse C, et al. Pharmacodynamic resistance to warfarin is associated with nucleotide substitutions in VKORC1. J Thromb Haemost. 2008;6(10):1663–70.

[106] Bodin L, Perdu J, Diry M, Horellou M-H, Loriot M-A. Multiple genetic alterations in vitamin K epoxide reductase complex subunit 1 gene (VKORC1) can explain the high dose requirement during oral anticoagulation in humans. J Thromb Haemost. 2008;6(8): 1436–9.

[107] Peoc'h K, Pruvot S, Gourmel C, Dit Sollier CB, Drouet L. A new VKORC1 mutation leading to an isolated resistance to fluindione. Br J Haematol. 2009;145(6): 841–3.

[108] Harrington DJ, Siddiq S, Allford SL, Shearer MJ, Mumford AD. More on: Endoplasmic reticulum loop VKORC1 substitutions cause warfarin resistance but do not diminish

gamma-carboxylation of the vitamin K-dependent coagulation factors. J Thromb Haemost. 2011;9(5):1093–5.

[109] D'Andrea G, D'Ambrosio RL, Perna PD, Chetta M, Santacroce R, Brancaccio V, et al. A polymorphism in the VKORC1 gene is associated with an interindividual variability in the dose-anticoagulant effect of warfarin. Blood. 2005;105(2):645–9.

[110] Loebstein R, Dvoskin I, Halkin H, Vecsler M, Lubetsky A, Rechavi G, et al. A coding VKORC1 Asp36Tyr polymorphism predisposes to warfarin resistance. Blood. 2007;109(6):2477–80.

[111] Anton AI, Cerezo-Manchado JJ, Padilla J, Perez-Andreu V, Corral J, Vicente V, et al. Novel associations of VKORC1 variants with higher acenocoumarol requirements. PLoS One. 2013;8(5):e64469.

[112] Shuen AY, Wong BYL, Fu L, Selby R, Cole DEC. Evaluation of the warfarin-resistance polymorphism, VKORC1 Asp36Tyr, and its effect on dosage algorithms in a genetically heterogeneous anticoagulant clinic. Clin Biochem. 2012;45(6):397–401.

[113] Schmeits PCJ, Hermans MHA, Van Geest-Daalderop JHH, Poodt J, De Sauvage Nolting PRW, Conemans JMH. VKORC1 mutations in patients with partial resistance to phenprocoumon. Br J Haematol. 2010;148(6):955–7.

[114] Wilms EB, Touw DJ, Conemans JMH, Veldkamp R, Hermans M. A new VKORC1 allelic variant (p.Trp59Arg) in a patient with partial resistance to acenocoumarol and phenprocoumon. J Thromb Haemost. 2008;6(7):1224–6.

[115] Osman A, Enström C, Arbring K, Söderkvist P, Lindahl TL. Main haplotypes and mutational analysis of vitamin K epoxide reductase (VKORC1) in a Swedish population: A retrospective analysis of case records. J Thromb Haemost. 2006;4(8): 1723–9.

[116] Bodin L, Horellou MH, Flaujac C, Loriot MA, Samama MM. A vitamin K epoxide reductase complex subunit-1 (VKORC1) mutation in a patient with vitamin K antagonist resistance. J Thromb Haemost. 2005;3(7):1533–5.

[117] Moreau C, Bajolle F, Siguret V, Loriot M-A, Bonnet D. Genetic resistance to warfarin therapy masked by amiodarone in a 2-year-old girl with mitral valve replacement. J Thromb Haemost. 2013;11(3):555–72.

[118] Orsi FA, Annichino Bizzacchi JM, de Paula EV, Ozelo MC, Langley MR, Weck KE. VKORC1 V66M mutation in African Brazilian patients resistant to oral anticoagulant therapy. Thromb Res. 2010;126(3):e206–10.

[119] Greaves J. Warfarin-resistant rats. R Soc Health J. 1970;90(6):289.

[120] Greaves JH. Resistance to anticoagulants in rodents. Pestic Sci. 1971;2(6):276–9.

[121] Lund M. Resistance to warfarin in the common Rat. Nature. 1964;203(4946):778.

[122] Lund M. Resistance of rodents to rodenticides. World Rev Pest Control. 1967;6(4):131–8.

[123] Jackson WB, Kaukeinen D. Resistance of wild Norway rats in North Carolina to warfarin rodenticide. Science. 1972;176(4041):1343–4.

[124] Jackson WB, Ashton AD. Case histories of anticoagulant resistance. In: Pesticide Resistance: Strategies and Tactics for Management. Washington, D.C.: National Academies Press; 1986.

[125] Rost S, Pelz H-J, Menzel S, MacNicoll AD, León V, Song K-J, et al. Novel mutations in the VKORC1 gene of wild rats and mice – a response to 50 years of selection pressure by warfarin? BMC Genet. 2009;10:4.

[126] Pelz H-J, Rost S, Hünerberg M, Fregin A, Heiberg A-C, Baert K, et al. The genetic basis of resistance to anticoagulants in rodents. Genetics. 2005;170(4):1839–47.

[127] Runge M, von Keyserlingk M, Braune S, Becker D, Plenge-Bönig A, Freise JF, et al. Distribution of rodenticide resistance and zoonotic pathogens in Norway rats in Lower Saxony and Hamburg, Germany. Pest Manag Sci. 2013;69(3):403–8.

[128] Grandemange A, Lasseur R, Longin-Sauvageon C, Benoit E, Berny P. Distribution of VKORC1 single nucleotide polymorphism in wild Rattus norvegicus in France. Pest Manag Sci. 2010;66(3):270–6.

[129] Buckle A. Anticoagulant resistance in the United Kingdom and a new guideline for the management of resistant infestations of Norway rats (Rattus norvegicus Berk.). Pest Manag Sci. 2013;69(3):334–41.

[130] Haniza MZH, Adams S, Jones EP, MacNicoll A, Mallon EB, Smith RH, et al. Large-scale structure of brown rat (*Rattus norvegicus*) populations in England: Effects on rodenticide resistance. Peer J. 2015;3:e1458.

[131] Berny P, Fourel I, Lattard V. Anticoagulant rodenticides: Resistance and residues in Norway rats in France. Vertebr Pest Conf. 2014;342–6.

[132] Pelz H-J. Resistance-problems in control of rats and house mice with anticoagulants. Gesunde Pflanz Ger FR. 1990;42(12):435.

[133] Pelz H-J, Rost S, Müller E, Esther A, Ulrich RG, Müller CR. Distribution and frequency of VKORC1 sequence variants conferring resistance to anticoagulants in Mus musculus. Pest Manag Sci. 2012;68(2):254–9.

[134] Goulois J, Chapuzet A, Lambert V, Chatron N, Tchertanov L, Legros L, et al. Evidence of a target resistance to antivitamin K rodenticides in the roof rat Rattus rattus: Identification and characterisation of a novel Y25F mutation in the VKORC1 gene. Pest Manag Sci. 2016;72(3):544–50.

[135] Matagrin B, Hodroge A, Montagut-Romans A, Andru J, Fourel I, Besse S, et al. New insights into the catalytic mechanism of vitamin K epoxide reductase (VKORC1) – The

catalytic properties of the major mutations of rVKORC1 explain the biological cost associated to mutations. FEBS Open Biol. 2013;3:144–50.

[136] Greaves JH, Ayres P. Warfarin resistance and vitamin K requirement in the rat. Lab Anim. 1973;7(2):141–8.

[137] Markussen MD, Heiberg A-C, Nielsen R, Leirs H. Vitamin K requirement in Danish anticoagulant-resistant Norway rats (Rattus norvegicus). Pest Manag Sci. 2003;59(8): 913–20.

[138] Kohn MH, Price RE, Pelz H-J. A cardiovascular phenotype in warfarin-resistant VKORC1 mutant rats. Artery Res. 2008;2(4):138–47.

[139] Markussen MD, Heiberg A-C, Fredholm M, Kristensen M. Differential expression of cytochrome P450 genes between bromadiolone-resistant and anticoagulant-susceptible Norway rats: A possible role for pharmacokinetics in bromadiolone resistance. Pest Manag Sci. 2008;64(3):239–48.

[140] Ishizuka M, Okajima F, Tanikawa T, Min H, Tanaka KD, Sakamoto KQ, et al. Elevated warfarin metabolism in warfarin-resistant roof rats (rattus rattus) in Tokyo. Drug Metab Dispos. 2007;35(1):62–6.

[141] Sugano S, Kobayashi T, Tanikawa T, Kawakami Y, Kojima H, Nakamura K, et al. Suppression of CYP3A2 mRNA expression in the warfarin-resistant roof rat, Rattus rattus: Possible involvement of cytochrome P450 in the warfarin resistance mechanism. Xenobiotica. 2001;31(7):399–407.

Chapter 3

The Risk Factors of Thrombogenic, Thrombophilia, and the Principle for Heparin Prophylaxis in Personalized Medicine

Andrey Momot, Irina Taranenko, Lyudmila Tsyvkina, Nadezhda Semenova and Irina Molchanova

Additional information is available at the end of the chapter

http://dx.doi.org/10.5772/64118

Abstract

This chapter presents new views on thrombogenic risk factors, thrombophilia, and thrombotic state of readiness preceding the thrombus formation. The modern methods of laboratory diagnostics of thrombotic state of readiness are considered to initiate thromboprophylaxis in patients irrespective of the presence of thrombophilia, as well as certain thrombogenic risk factors.

Keywords: venous thromboembolism, thrombogenic risk factors, thrombophilia, heparin prophylaxis

1. Introduction

One of the most important problems in modern medicine, which has interdisciplinary significance is venous thromboembolism prophylaxis or VTE (deep vein thrombosis, DVT, and pulmonary embolism, PE). This problem is associated with the high incidence of VTE around the world, with a direct connection of this pathology to the disablement and mortality of people, including those who underwent different invasive interventions and injuries (trauma, surgery, delivery) [1–7].

The association of tendency to thrombus formation with pregnancy complications and fetal death syndrome is equally significant [8, 9]. This phase of women's life is characterized with blood coagulation activation related to physiological pregnancy and it progresses through gestation. Its rationale is associated with the need to reduce blood loss during delivery. However, carrying of a pregnancy and the postpartum period are determined as confirmed risk factors for venous thrombosis and pulmonary embolism with the incidence being 4–50 times higher than in non-pregnant women [10–12].

Besides the reduction of the survival rate of VTE and concomitant post-thrombotic syndrome, it significantly shortens quality of life. The risk increases by 17 times after suffering from venous thrombosis [13]. However, a 20-year cumulative incidence of post-thrombotic syndrome after proximal deep vein thrombosis are about 40%.

Given the grandness of VTE for patients' life, many researchers aimed not only at improving methods of diagnostics and treatment of VTE (which is very crucial) but also at their anticipatory prophylaxis, prevention of primary or recurrent thrombotic events which is evidenced by the international study, ENDORSE (Epidemiologic International Day for the Evaluation of Patients at Risk of Venous Thrombosis in Acute Hospital Care Setting) [14].

Issues relating to thromboprophylaxis are represented in a number of national or international guidelines on the prevention and treatment of VTE based on the intercenter research and defining a standard tactic for thromboprophylaxis in obstetrics, oncology, cardiology, traumatology and orthopedics, neurosurgery, urology, thermal injury, and also in patients at high thrombogenic risk [15–21].

These are important, many-sided consolidated documents, which determine the modern level of knowledge on this issue. However, their structure involves such risk factors as peculiarities of scheduled operation and the type of anesthesia, a history of thrombosis, and inherited or acquired likelihood to thrombosis for specific laboratory parameters. Anyway, these features discussed in the documents, from the standpoint of evidence-based medicine, are relatively significant for the prediction of risk for thrombosis and do not always answer the following important questions: the rationale behind the prescription of anticoagulants in a specific patient, optimal dosage, and the required duration of their use.

The modern practice of anticoagulant prescription still consider low molecular weight heparin (LMWH) as a "gold standard" for the prevention of thrombosis in pregnancy, cancer, and postoperative thromboprophylaxis [17, 22] even though the whole group of new oral anticoagulants is used more often. Along with it, the discussion on the rationale behind laboratory monitoring of anticoagulant effects from the stand point of safety of used doses is continued and the determination of the effectiveness of the performed treatment that is presented in the review by Hassouna [23].

Besides, there is an equivocal interpretation of concepts directly related to VTE, such as thrombogenic risk factor, thrombophilia, and hypercoagulable state/syndrome, which disorient clinicians who wish to understand the problem.

The objective of this chapter is to find the perspective approaches for diagnostic and consultative assistance of patients with VTE. These approaches will involve the definition of thrombophilia and thrombogenic risk factors, as well as the state of thrombotic readiness when considering the advisability of heparin prophylaxis from the view point of personalized medicine.

Most people, who are permanent or temporary carriers or are at risk of thrombosis, do not suffer from thrombosis throughout their life, although they are likely to develop this disease [24, 25]. However, the presence of thrombogenic risk factors is often compared with thrombophilia, which leads to the over diagnosis of thrombophilia, especially during pregnancy and concomitant polypragmasy.

2. Modern perspective on thrombophilia

The attention of many researchers has always been on the possible causes and conditions in which thrombosis occurred. The risk of thrombosis is associated with trauma and surgical routines in the area of large venous lines (hip surgery, pelvic organ surgery), with other types of pathology and conditions which are predisposed to venous thrombosis (malignant tumors, obesity, diabetes, heart failure, prolonged immobilization, etc.) accompanied by the activation of blood coagulation. Taking this into consideration, in 1884, Rudolf Virchow reported that venous thrombosis are the result of the presence of, at least, one of the three basic factors, including (1) stasis of blood in lower extremity veins, (2) increased ability of blood to thrombus formation—we understand it as thrombotic state of readiness, and (3) damaged vessel walls [26]. It was determined that all the risk factors for venous thrombosis are carried out by these important pathophysiological processes and that VTE, in their absence, does not usually develop. In 1995, 30 years after the message of Egeberg (1965) [27] about the hereditary deficiency of antithrombin III, the World Health Organization and the International Society on Thrombosis and Hemostasis (ISTH) introduced the concept of thrombophilia as a state with an unusual tendency to result in thrombosis with early age onset, burden family history, severity of the thrombosis disproportionate to the known causal factors, and the presence of thrombosis recurrence [28]. The emphasis was made on the types of congenital thrombophilia associated with antithrombin III deficiency, factor V Leiden mutation (1691 G>A), prothrombin mutation (20210 G>A), and decreased levels of protein C and S. On the other hand, only the carriage of antiphospholipid antibodies in antiphospholipid syndrome (APS) associated with both arterial and venous thrombosis as well as with a miscarriage is considered to be an acquired thrombophilia.

In 2008, the version of the clinical practice recommended by the American College of Chest Physicians (ACCP) on antithrombotic and thrombolytic therapy was published, it identified thrombophilia as the presence of one or more of the following features, which included antithrombin deficiency, protein C or S deficiency, APS resistance (factor Va resistance to inactivate protein C), factor V Leiden mutation, prothrombin mutation (G20210A), hyperhomocysteinemia, homozygous carriers of heat-labile variant of methylenetetrahydrofolate reductase (MTHFR), the presence of antiphospholipid antibodies (aPL; lupus anticoagulant, β_2-glycoprotein I antibodies, or anticardiolipin antibodies) the increase in activity of factor VIII, a reduced level of protein Z [29].

In 2013, the International Consensus Statement, Prevention and Treatment of Venous Thromboembolism (guidelines according to scientific evidence) was published [15], where thrombophilia was determined as inherited or acquired state which shifts hemostatic balance toward hypercoagulation, characterized by the predisposition to the first episode of VTE and high risk of recurrence (**Table 1**).

Inherited thrombophilia	Acquired thrombophilia	Thrombophilia of mixed or unknown origin
Antithrombin deficiency	Acquired deficiency of	High levels of factor VIII
Protein C deficiency	natural coagulation inhibitors	High levels of factor IX
Protein S deficiency	Antiphospholipid syndrome	High levels of factor XI
Factor V Leiden	Myeloproliferative disease and	High levels of fibrinogen
Prothrombin 20210A	the presence of mutation JAK2V617F	High levels of TAFI
Disfibrinogenemia	Paroxysmal nocturnal hemoglobinuria	Low levels of TFPI
Factor XIII 34val		Factor V resistance to APC in the absence of FVL
Fibrinogen (G) 10034T		Hyperhomocysteinemia
Non-O blood type		High levels of PCI (PAI-3)
JAK 2		
Factor IX Padua		

Notes: TAFI—thrombin activated fibrinolysis inhibitor, TFPI—tissue factor pathway inhibitor, PCI—protein C inhibitor, PAI-3—plasminogen-activator inhibitor-3, FVL—Factor V Leiden, JAK 2—Janus kinase 2.

Table 1. Classification of hemostatic disorders associated with VTE according to their origin.

Risk factors	Odds ratio	95% CI
Increases body mass index (BMI) by 15 kg/m^2	1.08	1.05–1.11
Major surgery	18.95	9.22–38.97
Hospitalization for medical emergency	5.07	3.12–8.23
Trauma or fracture	4.56	2.46–8.46
Active malignancy	14.64	7.73–27.73
Neurological disease with the significant decrease in mobility	6.10	1.97–18.89
Pregnancy and postpartum period	4.24	1.30–13.84
Estrogen oral contraceptives	4.03	1.83–8.89
Hormonal replacement therapy in women	1.81	1.06–3.09

Note: CI—confidential interval.Data from Ref. [12].

Table 2. Independent risk factors for deep vein thrombosis and pulmonary embolism.

It is evident that peculiarities and clinical types of pathology mentioned in the table do not involve many other causes predisposing to thrombosis, which also promote the development of VTE—age, family or individual thrombotic history (e.g., after splenectomy), obesity, dislipidemy, the use of venous catheter, pregnancy, the postpartum period, administration of contraceptives containing estrogen, severe injury or surgery, hypodynamia, physical and psychological stress, active cancer, infection, autoimmune disorders, chronic heart failure, diabetes mellitus, varicose disease of the lower extremities, dehydration, and many others. These causes and their significance for the development of VTE were considerably described in the fundamental work by Heit [12], based on the earlier work of the author [30], as well as on the research by Barsoum et al. [31] (**Table 2**).

Considering this question, attention can be paid to the determination of clinical significance of some risk factors predisposing VTE, in accordance with recent guidelines of the European Society of Cardiology [17] (**Table 3**).

No	Measure of significance	Conditions promoting thromboembolism
1.	Significant risk factors (OR > 10)	Clot detachment; the first 3 months after hospitalization with HF/AF; prosthetics of lower extremities, a heavy injury, the first 3 months after MI; prior venous thromboembolic complications
2.	Moderate risk factors (OR = 2–9)	Arthroscopic surgery; autoimmune diseases; hemotransfusion; chemotherapy; congestive HF/PHD; HRT; malignant tumor; oral contraceptives; thrombophilia; stroke in anamnesis
3.	Weak risk factors (OR < 2)	Bed rest > 3 days; diabetes; arterial hypertension; long travel; age; laparoscopic surgery; obesity; pregnancy; varicose vein disease

Notes: OR—odds ratio, HF—heart failure, AF—atrial fibrillation, MI—myocardial infarction, PHD—pulmonary heart disease, HRT—hormone replacement therapy.

Table 3. Gradation of the risk factors for venous thromboembolic complications in cardiac patients.

Thus, it can be observed that there are no significant differences between thrombogenic risk factors and thrombophilia in modern guidelines and recommendations.

3. The question about the definition of "thrombogenic risk factor" and "thrombophilia"

It is believed that thrombophilia precedes and accompanies thrombosis and fetal loss syndrome [11, 32–34]. However, some clinicians deny the importance of genetic predisposition to the development of thrombosis, observed in **Table 1**, which is explained by the fact that the connection between these phenomena is not always seen [35]. Indeed, the direct association might be questionable, as evidenced by a number of publications, including a retrospective family cohort study involving 723 first- and second-degree relatives of 150 patients with venous thrombosis. The collected data in this study present interesting information about the importance of thrombotic risk in patients with inherited defects in the physiological anticoagulation system, developability of which is relatively small. Thus, the cumulative lifetime likelihood of thrombosis occurrence (penetrance) among the carriers of the most common family thrombophilia (factor V Leiden mutation) is only about 10%.

It is also pointed out that the factor V Leiden mutation is not necessarily manifested by the increased levels of D-dimer, polymorphism genes involved in the methionine metabolism by hyperhomocysteinemia, and rare homozygote gene of plasminogen activator inhibitor type 1 (PAI-1), by the increased activity of PAI-1 and suppression of fibrinolytic reactions. These thrombotic events are made possible in the presence of some mentioned gene polymorphisms, but when and how far, cannot be predicted and it depends on additional risk factors in certain cases, for example, dehydration, distress, or pregnancy. In this regard, there is a view that thrombosis are multifactorial (complex) disease that occurs when a person with identified thrombophilia is exposed to additional risk factors associated with the disease, due to personal characteristics, or due to the external environment [12]. Thus, in accordance with the published data, the risk of VTE among carriers of the factor V Leiden mutation increases with in particular age; most cases occur at the age of 50–55 years [36–38]. The carriers of homozygous factor V Leiden mutation might have a higher risk under the influence of the environment or other genetic risk factors. The penetrance of thrombosis phenotype increases among patients with multiple genetic defects (e.g., concomitant deficiency of antithrombin, protein C or S). The same indicator depends on the clinical effects of acquired risk factors, such as the use of combined oral contraceptives, pregnancy, or surgery. In particular, the relative risk of the VTE among the carriers of heterozygous factor V Leiden mutation with estrogen contraceptives increases by 30 times [38, 39].

In general, the presence of inherited thrombophilia increases the risk of VTE by seven times [40]. At the same time, as earlier mentioned (see **Table 2**), a number of acquired thrombogenic risk factors (major surgery, endoprosthesis replacement of large joints, hospitalization due to medical emergency, active cancer, etc.) without combination with inherited thrombophilia have no less prognostic value for VTE occurrence.

Despite this important and interesting information, it is still not clear—the difference between thrombogenic risk factors and thrombophilia.

From our point of view to avoid confusion, separation of terms "thrombogenic risk factors" and "thrombophilia" can be based (in a similar way) on the example referring APS to thrombophilia.

According to the recommendations of the ISTH, adopted in Sapporo (1998) and Sydney (2006) [41], diagnosis of APS is believed to be reliable when, at least, one or more clinical manifestations of this pathology (vascular thrombosis, pregnancy failure) are combined with the results of special laboratory tests (effects of lupus anticoagulant, antiphospholipid antibodies in the diagnostic titer; **Table 4**).

Clinical criteria		Laboratory criteria	
1.	Vascular thrombosis	**1.**	Anticardiolipin antibodies
	- One or more cases of arterial and/or venous thrombosis or thrombosis of small vessels in any organ or tissue.		- The presence of isotypes IgG and IgM in high titers in two or more studies with an interval of not less than 12 weeks.
	- Thrombosis must be confirmed by Doppler examination or histologically.		- Identifying antibodies IgG, IgM to β_2-glycoprotein I by a standardized ELISA test.
	- There should be morphologically symptoms of thrombosis without significant inflammation of vessel walls.	**2.**	Lupus anticoagulant
			- It is found in two or more consecutive tests with an interval of not less than 12 weeks
2.	Pregnancy failure		
	- Three or more unexplained cases of miscarriage up to 10 weeks of gestation excluding anatomic, genetic, hormonal causes and chromosomal abnormalities;		
	- One or more cases of intrauterine death of a normal fetus after 10 weeks of gestation;		
	- One or more cases of premature birth of a fetus after less than 34 weeks of gestation occurring with evident fetoplacental insufficiency or severe gestosis		

Table 4. Diagnostic criteria for diagnosis of antiphospholipid syndrome.

We suggest an extension of this approach (involving the combination of certain thrombogenic risk factors with thrombosis or fetal loss syndrome) to the methodology of thrombophilia diagnostics. The presence of certain causes predisposing to thrombosis in patients without their clinical realization cannot be referred to as thrombophilia (**Figure 1**).

We consider that thrombophilia is essentially not a disease, but it is a pathological condition caused by a combination of risk factors, realized by the development of thrombosis (thromboses), which can be obtained according to the individual medical history. It may be inherited or associated with the disease (e.g., cancer), drug intake (e.g., oral contraceptives, erythropoiesis stimulating agents), or state of health (e.g., pregnancy, postpartum period). It is very important to understand and accept this position because susceptibility to the disease does not imply the presence of indications for primary or secondary prophylaxis or treatment [12].

In addition to APS, according to the same criteria, Trousseau's syndrome (migrating venous thrombosis in the presence of cancer procoagulant), Moschkowitz's syndrome (arterial microthrombosis on the background of circulation of large multimers of von Willebrand factor in blood, in the presence of metalloproteinase ADAMTS-13 deficiency), heparin-induced thrombocytopenia of 2 type—HIT-2 (subcutaneous and systemic venous thrombosis in the presence of antiheparin antibodies) and warfarin necrosis or Legg's disease on the background of inherited protein C deficiency can be referred to as thrombophilia. We consider that this list is not complete.

Thus, it is suggested:

1. Syndromic approach to the diagnostics of thrombophilia.
2. Identification of all causes promoting the development of VTE (including known states identified as thrombophilia) as thrombogenic risk factors.

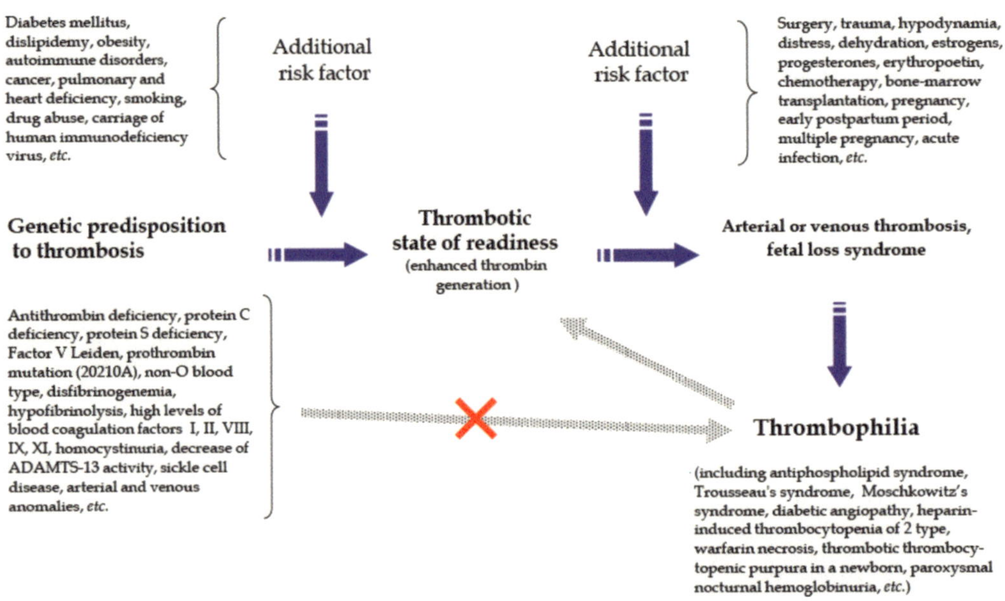

Figure 1. Hypothesis about the interaction of thrombogenic risk factors, thrombotic readiness, and thrombophilia in the development of thrombosis and fetal loss syndrome.

Presently, there are more than 100 variants of thrombophilia and various thrombogenic risk factors described, which are capable in their combination to lead to a vascular catastrophe [12, 42, 43]. However, it is believed as insufficient to divide them into hereditary (congenital) and acquired. From the point of view of personalized thromboprophylaxis, the classification of thrombogenic risk factors should be based on the duration of exposure to a human body and controllability by the patient or by means of modern medicine, to reduce the probability of VTE.

Uncontrollable risk factors, such as age, sex, family and personal thrombotic history, the carriage of thrombogenic mutations, non-O blood group, and several others, are not amenable to correction and accompany the person for life. The temporary and controllable risk factors are much more numerous, which, in turn, can be divided into, associated with lifestyle (e.g., bad habits, obesity, hypodynamia (including long flight), mental distress and physical overload, as well as dehydration during sporting activities), individual characteristics (pregnancy, postpartum period), caused by a disease (trauma, cancer, sepsis, myocardial infraction and stroke, diabetes, atherosclerosis, arterial hypertension, cardiac rhythm disorders, HIV infection), and iatrogenic—caused by surgery and prescription of some medicine with estrogen therapy, progesterone therapy, selective estrogen receptor modulators, chemotherapy, erythropoietin administration, in some cases with usage of heparin or coumarins.

Controllability of these risk factors is different and might be considered individually in all cases, from the point of view of both etiology and pathogenesis of thrombosis. If modern possibilities of medicine are limited to radical correction of risk factors existing for life or permanently, then, for example, substitution of deficiency of physiological anticoagulants, heparin prophylaxis, usage of folic acid with correction of elevated levels of homocysteine in blood, blood viscosity reduction during dehydration or erythrocytosis, and other types of pathogenetic therapy allow the modification of identified thrombogenic risk factors and a reduction in the probability of clinical manifestation of VTE.

Nowadays, the mentioned recommendations do not show the association between the presence of "thrombophilia", "thrombogenic risk factors", and blood coagulation activation for known laboratory markers. However, it can be suggested that blood coagulation activation is the main condition for thrombus formation and a prerequisite for heparin prophylaxis.

4. Thrombotic readiness

The terms "thrombophilia" and "hypercoagulability" are often considered by many authors as synonyms, but in real sense, these notions are different. Hypercoagulation or "hypercoagulation syndrome/state" is a laboratory phenomenon by which "in vitro" with the help of special methods of hemostasis system analysis platelet activation and the process of fibrin formation, and in some cases, inhibition of fibrinolytic reactions are recognized. Hypercoagulation can be promoted by drugs commonly used to treat bleeding in hemophilia, sepsis, inflammation, surgery, hemostasis, and atherosclerosis as well as by many other factors and conditions. However, it can appear in the analysis of hemostatic parameters—in the case of warfarin skin necrosis, associated with congenital protein C deficiency due to treatment with coumarins, heparin-induced thrombocytopenia with heparin prescription, and effects of lupus anticoagulant peculiar to antiphospholipid syndrome. Consequently, the notions such as "hypercoagulation syndrome" and "hypercoagulation state" do not meet the essence of the pathological process and should therefore be considered obsolete.

We proposed an alternative, a clinically justifiable notion of "the state of thrombotic readiness", which can combine laboratory detected hypercoagulation or hypocoagulation (in cases of APS,

HIT-2, warfarin necrosis, and others), increased levels of intravascular coagulation markers due to the excessive thrombin generation, and also a number of clinical signs of prethrombosis. Accordingly, a realization of this readiness with the continued risk factors and their multiplication (e.g., surgery, injury, inflammation, emergency, immobilization, heart failure, dehydration, distress, intake of estrogens, etc.) is manifested by the vascular catastrophe in **Figure 1**. Thus, the state of thrombotic readiness might be formed by cooperation of various thrombogenic risk factors and directly precedes thrombosis, and also accompanies it in its absence or the low efficiency of antithrombotic prophylaxis and therapy.

Based on the study of their functional activity (in an aggregometer or platelet function analyzer, PFA-100/PFA-200) or by increased expression of β-thrombomodulin, as well as III and IV platelet factors, platelet activation can be attributed to the laboratory markers of the state of thrombotic readiness. No less significant indicator of such readiness is the increase in concentrations of some coagulation activation markers and fibrinolysis —tissue factor (TF), activated factor VII, thrombin-antithrombin (TAT) complex, prothrombin fragment 1 + 2, fibrinopeptide A, soluble fibrin-monomer complexes, and D-dimers. The latter plays a special role, considering the experience of their wide use in clinical practice for the diagnosis of VTE and for monitoring the efficiency of anticoagulant use.

D-dimers are known to be as a result of the sequential influence of thrombin, activated factor XIII, and plasmin on fibrinogen [44–46]. The increase of D-dimer concentration is widely used in the diagnostics as a laboratory criterion for activation of hypercoagulation and fibrinolysis, under such human pathologies, as disseminated intravascular coagulation [47, 48], as well as deep vein thrombosis of the lower extremity and pulmonary embolism [49, 50]. This parameter is widely studied as a very effective step in the diagnostic algorithm for patients with suspected first episode of PE or DVT [51]. There are many publications on the specificity and sensitivity of this marker of hemostatic reactions for the diagnostics of VTE [52]. It should be noted that the negative value of D-dimer allows the exclusion of VTE due to its high sensitivity of about 95% [53].

Recent studies in this field involve diagnostic use of age-adjusted D-dimer cutoff levels in adult patients [17, 54]. To provide the most accurate diagnostics of VTE, besides D-dimer identification, it is suggested to take into account genetic susceptibility, inflammation, immune characteristics, hemodynamic factors, as well as epigenetics profile or circulating levels of microRNA [55–58]. In this regard, the role of biomarkers such as C-reactive protein, soluble P-selectin, coagulation factor VIII activity, microvesicle containing tissue factor and white blood cells as prospective candidates is considered [53, 59, 60]. The rationale behind the use of these markers to diagnose VTE (except, D-dimers) remains unclear.

However, in this work, we were interested in a different, but no less important question, which is not devoted to the diagnostics, but to the prevention of venous thrombosis—whose blood coagulation activation marker is more acceptable for decision making to initiate heparin prophylaxis and are used in case of confirmed VTE therapeutic doses of heparin. To find such methodological approach, we suggest a return to the mechanism of anticoagulant action of heparin and low molecular weight heparin (LMWH) analogues. Thrombin is a key enzyme of the blood coagulation system; it is also a vitamin K-dependent protein related to the serine protease class. In the liver, there is a synthesis of its precursor—prothrombin, which is further present in plasma and can be converted into α-thrombin by blood coagulation activation. This transformation occurs in composition of factors Xa, Va, and II on the surface of activated blood cell membranes and endothelium [61, 62]. LMWH is known to inhibit factors Xa and IIa (thrombin) with plasma antithrombin, as well as to promote TFPI expression [63]. The total result of these reactions is considered to be the decrease of high initial rate of thrombin generation, which should be achieved in patients with thrombotic state of readiness.

An excessive thrombin generation can be determined, for example, by calibrated automated thrombography (thrombin generation test, TGT) suggested by Hemker et al. [64, 65], which allows measuring the dynamics of the formation and inactivation of thrombin with improved accuracy. During thrombin generation test (with the use of fluorimeter and computer data processing), the area under the curve and the peak rate are measured having an ascending part, the area of achieving the maximum, and the descending part, which characterizes the inactivation of the enzyme. This test captures the end result of a complex array of enzymatic interactions involved in blood coagulation and reacts on any trend toward coagulation activation in blood plasma, as a result, it has integrated nature. According to the opinion of a number of authors [66–68], measurement of an individual's capacity to generate thrombin, which occur under the action of TF in vitro, may be a better indicator of blood coagulation activation, compared to tests designed to study fibrin clot formation or determine potential biomarkers—prothrombin fragment 1 + 2, fibrinopeptide A, TAT complex, and D-dimers.

Based on the opinion of other authors, we consider that excessive (related to reference interval) thrombin generation can be accepted not only for the identification of blood coagulation activation but also as an objective prerequisite for the prescription of prophylactic LMWH in certain cases. At the same time, according to the recent International Consensus Statement [15], prophylaxis of VTE in women with thrombophilia depends on the type of thrombophilia, and also on other risk factors, such as age 35 years or more, personal or family history of VTE, obesity, immobilization during pregnancy, multiparity, or gemellarity. Prophylaxis consist of clinical surveillance, elastic compression stockings, and/or LMWH administration. It is often decided on an individual basis, because randomized studies in this regard were not performed.

In contrast, to decide whether to use LMWH as thromboprophylaxis during pregnancy, we consider the possible use of objective laboratory criteria. For this purpose, in our center reference intervals, the dynamics of thrombin generation parameters were determined in the blood plasma of 301 women during physiological pregnancy (full text of the article is presented in the publication of 2016). This parameter was studied by means of flatbed fluorometer Fluoroskan Ascent (ThermoFisher SCIENTIFIC). Tissue factor was used as an activator of coagulation in a concentration of 5 pmol/l. Women were examined in a non-pregnant state, at different stages of physiological pregnancy (6–8, 12–13, 22–24, 34–36 weeks of gestation) and 2–3 days after vaginal delivery.

As a result, during pregnancy, the acceleration of a parameter time to reach peak thrombin (ttPeak) was determined in blood plasma, as well as changes of two other parameters used for the assessment of thrombin generation intensity–peak thrombin and endogenous thrombin potential (ETP, **Figure 2**). Since early pregnancy (6–8 weeks), the latter two parameters were on the increase (in comparison with pregravid period for peak thrombin by 55.1% and ETP by 39.6%) and correlated well with each other throughout pregnancy (Spearman correlation coefficient 0.80; $p < 0.001$).

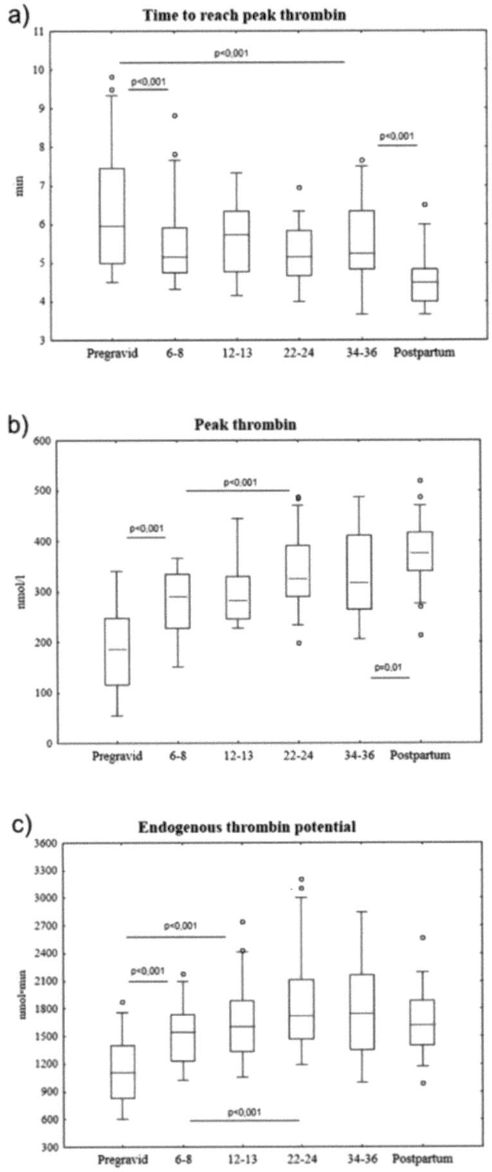

Figure 2. Box plots of reference intervals in pregravid period, at different stages of pregnancy, and in 2–3 days after spontaneous labor for (a) time to reach peak thrombin, (b) peak thrombin, and (c) endogenous thrombin potential. In figures, box plots represent the range of data from the 25th to 75th percentiles, while the bar in the middle of each box plot represents the median value obtained excluding outliers. Circles indicate outliers (1.5 × the interquartile range) and extreme values (3.0 × the interquartile range) outside the central box, respectively.

In our opinion, exceeding the upper values of peak thrombin and/or ETP at different stages of pregnancy can be considered as an objective prerequisite for the prescription of LMWHs, irrespective of the causes or known personal thrombogenic risk factors (carriage of factor V Leiden mutation, prothrombin mutation, deficiency of physiological anticoagulants, thrombotic history, and others). This approach was used for the initiation of heparin prophylaxis in women who conceived after in vitro fertilization cycle, as an extension of the study published earlier [69]. Another perspective research method for the assessment of thrombotic state of readiness is the assessment of spatial fibrin clot growth (thrombodynamics). This integrated method designed to study hemostatic system is based on the initiation of coagulation by means of plasma contact with immobilized TF and monitoring fibrin clot spreading from activating surface [70]. This method was widely used to study hemophilia, mechanisms of action of antihemophilic drugs, and the development of new ones [71, 72]. There are some data about the use of this method in pharmacology, such as the development of thrombin inhibitors [73], a study of their antidotes [74], or study of the procoagulant activity of microparticles [75]. Clinical studies of the capacity of thrombodynamics to identify the development of procoagulant states are presented by the studies of patients with sepsis [76]. Further development of this method (with the tentative title thrombodynamics 4D) has been presented in a number of studies [77, 78]. The approach, based on videomicroscopy of fluorescence, produced by thrombin-sensitive substrate, followed by a solution of an inverse reaction-diffusion problem, allows not only observation of spatial clot growth but also the determination of thrombin as a function of time and distance from the activator.

The appearance of these integrated methods represents undeniable progress in the field of diagnostic improvement of a wide range of hemostatic disorders. They can be used in the selection of risk group patients according to thrombotic and hemorrhagic complications, but it is necessary to consider that, as a rule, only platelet-, erythrocyte-, and leukocyte-poor plasma can be analyzed, which eliminates the influence of a blood cell component on the obtained results.

5. Conclusion

In conclusion of this chapter, the following summary can be made. Nowadays, highlighted thrombogenic risk factors in their prognostic value are often equal to different types of thrombophilia; based on this, their separation loses its sense. We consider that any cause promoting thrombus formation can be referred to as thrombogenic risk factors, which can manifest itself or not, by thrombosis in patients throughout life. We suggest referring those pathological states or syndromes, which manifested themselves as thrombotic events (e.g., antiphospholipid syndrome) to thrombophilia. It allows for a reduction in hyperdiagnostics of thrombophilia and identifying patients with thrombophilia and patients in need of secondary thromboprophylaxis, taking into account their identified thrombogenic risk factors. We consider that the presence of some thrombogenic risk factors, which have not manifested themselves by thrombosis, is not a safe prerequisite for medicamental thromboprophylaxis. From the point of view of personalized medicine, controllable risk factors should be identified in patients with the aim of elimination or modification, thereby reducing the likelihood of thrombosis. On the other hand, the presence of enhanced thrombin generation or excessive fibrin formation (in thrombodynamics test) among the manifestations of thrombotic state of readiness can be referred to as objective reasons for the prescription of anticoagulants.

We hope that a consideration of the proposed approaches to the diagnostics of thrombophilia and thromboprophylaxis will promote further development of preventative direction in this field of medicine.

Acknowledgements

The authors greatly appreciate the help of Gulnara Chueva and Anastasia Sidorenko in the preparation of this chapter for publication.

Author details

Andrey Momot[1*], Irina Taranenko[1], Lyudmila Tsyvkina[1], Nadezhda Semenova[2] and Irina Molchanova[2]

*Address all correspondence to: xyzan@yandex.ru

1 Altai Branch of FSFI "National Research Center for Hematology" of Ministry of Healthcare of the Russian Federation, Barnaul, Russia

2 Clinical Regional Hospital, Barnaul, Russia

References

[1] Cohen AT, Agnelli G, Anderson FA, Arcelus JI, Bergqvist D, Brecht JG, Greer IA, Heit JA, Hutchinson JL, Kakkar AK, Mottier D, Oger E, Samama MM, Spannagl M; VTE Impact Assessment Group in Europe (VITAE). Venous thromboembolism (VTE) in Europe. The number of VTE events and associated morbidity and mortality. Thromb Haemost. 2007;98:756–764. DOI: 10.1160/TH07-03-0212

[2] Go AS, Mozaffarian D, Roger VL, Benjamin EJ, Berry JD, Blaha MJ, Dai S, Ford ES, Fox CS, Franco S, Fullerton HJ, Gillespie C, Hailpern SM, Heit JA, Howard VJ, Huffman MD, Judd SE, Kissela BM, Kittner SJ, Lackland DT, Lichtman JH, Lisabeth LD, Mackey RH, Magid DJ, Marcus GM, Marelli A, Matchar DB, McGuire DK, Mohler ER 3rd, Moy CS, Mussolino ME, Neumar RW, Nichol G, Pandey DK, Paynter NP, Reeves MJ, Sorlie PD, Stein J, Towfighi A, Turan TN, Virani SS, Wong ND, Woo D, Turner MB; American Heart

Association Statistics Committee and Stroke Statistics Subcommittee. Heart disease and stroke statistics – 2014 update: a report from the American Heart Association. Circulation. 2014;129:e28–e292. DOI: 10.1161/01.cir.0000441139.02102.80

[3] Silverstein MD, Heit JA, Mohr DN, Petterson TM, O'Fallon WM, Melton LJ. 3rd. Trends in the incidence of deep vein thrombosis and pulmonary embolism: a 25-year population-based study. Arch Intern Med. 1998;158:585–593. DOI: 10.1001/archinte.158.6.585.

[4] Frank B, Ariza L, Lamparter H, Grossmann V, Prochaska JH, Ullmann A, Kindler F, Weisser G, Walter U, Lackner KJ, Espinola-Klein C, Münzel T, Konstantinides SV, Wild PS; VTEval study group. Rationale and design of three observational, prospective cohort studies including biobanking to evaluate and improve diagnostics, management strategies and risk stratification in venous thromboembolism: the VTEval Project. BMJ Open. 2015;5:e008157. DOI: 10.1136/bmjopen-2015-008157

[5] White RH. The epidemiology of venous thromboembolism. Circulation. 2003;107:4I–8I. DOI: 10.1161/01.cir.0000078468.11849.66

[6] Pengo V, Lensing AW, Prins MH, Marchiori A, Davidson BL, Tiozzo F, Albanese P, Biasiolo A, Pegoraro C, Iliceto S, Prandoni P. for the Thromboembolic Pulmonary Hypertension Study Group. Incidence of chronic thromboembolic pulmonary hypertension after pulmonary embolism. N Engl J Med. 2004;350:2257–2264. DOI: 10.1056/nejmoa032274

[7] Lefebvre P, Laliberté F, Nutescu EA, Duh MS, LaMori J, Bookhart BK, Olson WH, Dea K, Schein J, Kaatz S. All-cause and potentially disease-related health care costs associated with venous thromboembolism in commercial, Medicare, and Medicaid beneficiaries. J Manag Care Pharm. 2012;18:363–374.

[8] Brenner B. Haemostatic changes in pregnancy. Thromb Res. 2004;114:409–414. DOI: 10.1016/j.thromres.2004.08.004

[9] Franchini M. Haemostasis and pregnancy. Thromb Haemost. 2006;95:401–413. DOI: 10.1160/th05-11-0753

[10] Brenner BR, Nowak-Göttl U, Kosch A, Manco-Johnson M, Laposata M. Diagnostic studies for thrombophilia in women on hormonal therapy and during pregnancy, and in children. Arch Pathol Lab Med. 2002;126:1296–1303.

[11] Braekkan SK, Mathiesen EB, Njølstad I, Wilsgaard T, Hansen JB. Hematocrit and risk of venous thromboembolism in a general population. The Tromso study. Haematologica. 2010;95:270–275. DOI: 10.3324/haematol.2009.008417

[12] Heit J. Thrombophilia: Clinical and Laboratory Assessment and Management. In: Kithens CS, Kessler CM, Konkle BA, editors. Consultative Hemostasis and Thrombosis. 3rd ed. Philadelphia: ELSEVIER Saunders; 2013. pp. 205–239. DOI: 10.1016/B978-1-4557-2296-9.00014-2

[13] Heit JA, Melton LJ 3rd, Lohse CM, Petterson TM, Silverstein MD, Mohr DN, O'Fallon WM. Incidence of venous thromboembolism in hospitalized patients vs community residents. Mayo Clin Proc. 2001;76:1102–1110. DOI: 10.4065/76.11.1102

[14] Cohen AT, Tapson VF, Bergmann JF, Goldhaber SZ, Kakkar AK, Deslandes B, Huang W, Zayaruzny M, Emery L, Anderson FA Jr; ENDORSE Investigators. Venous thromboembolism risk and prophylaxis in acute hospital care setting (ENDORSE study): a multinational cross-sectional study. Lancet. 2008;371:387–394. DOI: 10.1016/S0140-6736(08)60202-0.

[15] Balas P, Nicolaides A, editors. Thrombophilia. Prevention and treatment of venous thromboembolism. International Consensus Statement (Guidelines according to scientific evidence). Int Angiol. 2013;32:188–200.

[16] Langford Nj, Stansby G, Avital L. The management of venous thromboembolic diseases and the role of thrombophilia testing: summary of NICE Guideline CG144. Acute Med. 2012;11:138–142.

[17] Konstantinides SV, Torbicki A, Agnelli G, Danchin N, Fitzmaurice D, Galiè N, Gibbs JS, Huisman MV, Humbert M, Kucher N, Lang I, Lankeit M, Lekakis J, Maack C, Mayer E, Meneveau N, Perrier A, Pruszczyk P, Rasmussen LH, Schindler TH, Svitil P, Vonk Noordegraaf A, Zamorano L, Zompatori M; Task Force for the Diagnosis and Management of Acute Pulmonary Embolism of the European Society of Cardiology (ESC). 2014 ESC guidelines on the diagnosis and management of acute pulmonary embolism. Eur Heart J. 2014;35:3033–3069, 3069a–3069k. DOI: 10.1093/eurheartj/ehu283

[18] Tait C, Baglin T, Watson H, Laffan M, Makris M, Perry D, Keeling D; British Committee for Standards in Haematology. Guidelines on the investigation and management of venous thrombosis at unusual sites. Br J Haematol. 2012;159:28–38. DOI: 10.1111/j.1365-2141.2012.09249.x

[19] Lyman GH, Khorana AA, Kuderer NM, Lee AY, Arcelus JI, Balaban EP, Clarke JM, Flowers CR, Francis CW, Gates LE, Kakkar AK, Key NS, Levine MN, Liebman HA, Tempero MA, Wong SL, Prestrud AA, Falanga A; American Society of Clinical Oncology Clinical Practice. Venous thromboembolism prophylaxis and treatment in patients with cancer: American Society of Clinical Oncology clinical practice guideline update. J Clin Oncol. 2013;31:2189–2204. DOI: 10.1200/jco.2013.49.1118

[20] James A; Committee on Practice Bulletins-Obstetrics. Practice bulletin no. 123: thromboembolism in pregnancy. Obstet Gynecol. 2011;118:718–729. DOI: 10.1097/AOG.0b013e3182310c4c.

[21] Heffner JE. Update of antithrombotic guidelines: medical professionalism and the funnel of knowledge. Chest. 2016;149:293–294. DOI: 10.1016/j.chest.2015.12.005.

[22] Cohen AT, Imfeld S, Rider T. Phase III trials of new oral anticoagulants in the acute treatment and secondary prevention of VTE: comparison and critique of study methodology and results. Adv Ther. 2014;31:473–493. DOI: 10.1007/s12325-014-0119-7.

[23] Hassouna H. Thrombophilia and hypercoagulability. Med Princ Pract. 2009;18:429–440. DOI: 10.1159/000235891.

[24] Bovill EG, Hasstedt SJ, Leppert MF, Long GL. Hereditary thrombophilia as a model for multigenic disease. Thromb Haemost. 1999;82:662–666.

[25] Makris M. Thrombophilia: grading the risk. Blood. 2009;113:5038–5039. DOI: 10.1182/blood-2009-02-203281.

[26] Virchow R. Neuer fall von todlicher emboli der lungenarterie. Arch Pathol Anat. 1856;10:225–228. DOI: 10.1007/bf01933614

[27] Egeberg O. Inherited antithrombin deficiency causing thrombophilia. Thromb Diath Haemorrh. 1965;13:516–530.

[28] WHO: Inherited thrombophilia: report of a joint WHO/International Society of Thrombosis and Haemostasis (ISTH) Meeting. Geneva, World Health Organization. 1995.

[29] Bates SM, Greer IA, Pabinger I, Sofaer S, Hirsh J; American College of Chest Physicians. Venous thromboembolism, thrombophilia, antithrombotic therapy, and pregnancy: American College of Chest Physicians evidence-based clinical practice guidelines (8th Edition). Chest. 2008;133:844S–886S. DOI: 10.1378/chest.08-0761.

[30] Heit JA, Silverstein MD, Mohr DN, Petterson TM, O'Fallon WM, Melton LJ 3rd. Risk factors for deep vein thrombosis and pulmonary embolism: a population-based case-control study. Arch Intern Med. 2000;160:809–815.

[31] Barsoum MK, Heit JA, Ashrani AA, Leibson CL, Petterson TM, Bailey KR. Is progestin an independent risk factor for incident venous thromboembolism? A population-based case-control study. Thromb Res. 2010;126:373–378. DOI: 10.1016/j.thromres.2010.08.010.

[32] Bonnar J. Hypercoagulable States and Pregnancy. In: Seghatchian M, Samama M, Hecker SP, editors. Hypercoagulable states: fundamental aspects, acquired disorders, and congenital thrombophilia. Boca Raton, New York, London, Tokyo: CRS Press Inc.; 1996. pp. 253–257.

[33] Christiansen SC, Cannegieter SC, Koster T, Vandenbroucke JP, Rosendaal FR. Thrombophilia, clinical factors, and recurrent venous thrombotic events. JAMA. 2005;293:2352–2361.

[34] Geerts W, Pineo G, Heit J, Bergqvist D, Lassen MR, Colwell CW, Ray JG. Prevention of venosus thromboembolism: the seventh ACCP conference on antithrombotic therapy. Chest. 2004;126:338S–400S.

[35] Martinelli I, Manucci PM, De Stefano V, Taioli E, Rossi V, Crosti F, Paciaroni K, Leone G, Faioni EM. Different risks of thrombosis in four coagulation defects associated with inherited thrombophilia: a study of 150 families. Blood. 1998;92:2353–2358.

[36] Rosendaal FR, Vessey M, Rumley A, Daly E, Woodward M, Helmerhorst FM, Lowe GD. Hormonal replacement therapy, prothrombotic mutations and the risk of venous thrombosis. Br J Haematol. 2002;116:851–854.

[37] Cushman M, Kuller LH, Prentice R, Rodabough RJ, Psaty BM, Stafford RS, Sidney S, Rosendaal FR; Women's Health Initiative Investigators. Estrogen plus progestin and risk of venous thrombosis. JAMA. 2004;292:1573–1580.

[38] Wu O, Robertson L, Langhorne P, Twaddle S, Lowe GD, Clark P, Greaves M, Walker ID, Brenkel I, Regan L, Greer IA. Oral contraceptives, hormone replacement therapy, thrombophilias and risk of venous thromboembolism: a systematic review. The Thrombosis: Risk and Economic Assessment of Thrombophilia Screening (TREATS) Study. Thromb Haemost. 2005;94:17–25.

[39] van Vlijmen EF, Veeger NJ, Middeldorp S, Hamulyák K, Prins MH, Büller HR, Meijer K. Thrombotic risk during oral contraceptive use and pregnancy in women with factor V Leiden or prothrombin mutation: a rational approach to contraception. Blood. 2011;118:2055–2061. DOI: 10.1182/blood-2011-03-345678.

[40] Mahmoodi BK, Brouwer JL, Ten Kate MK, Lijfering WM, Veeger NJ, Mulder AB, Kluin-Nelemans HC, Van Der Meer J. A prospective cohort study on the absolute risks of venous thromboembolism and predictive value of screening asymptomatic relatives of patients with hereditary deficiencies of protein S, protein C or antithrombin. J Thromb Haemost. 2010; 8:1193–1200. DOI: 10.1111/j.1538-7836.2010.03840.x.

[41] Harris E, Pierangeli S. Primary, secondary and catastrophic antiphospholipid syndrome: what's in a name. Semin Thromb Hemost. 2008;34:219–226. DOI: 10.1055/s-0028-1082265.

[42] Douketis JD, Spyropoulos AC, Spencer FA, Mayr M, Jaffer AK, Eckman MH, Dunn AS, Kunz R; American College of Chest Physicians. Perioperative management of antithrombotic therapy: antithrombotic therapy and prevention of thrombosis, 9th ed: American College of Chest Physicians evidence-based clinical practice guidelines. Chest. 2012;141:326S–350S. DOI: 10.1378/chest.11-2298.

[43] Prandoni P. Acquired risk factors for venous thromboembolism in medical patients. Hematology. 2005;458–461.

[44] Uchikova EH, Ledjev II. Changes in haemostasis during normal pregnancy. Eur J Obstet Gynecol Reprod Biol. 2005;119:185–188.

[45] Eichinger S. D-dimer testing in pregnancy. Semin Vasc Med. 2005;5:375–378.

[46] Kline J, Williams G, Hernandez-Nino J. D-dimer concentrations in normal pregnancy: new diagnostic thresholds are needed. Clin Chem. 2005;51:825–829.

[47] Toh CH, Hoots WK; SSC on Disseminated Intravascular Coagulation of the ISTH. The scoring system of the Scientific and Standardisation Committee on Disseminated

Intravascular Coagulation of the International Society on Thrombosis and Haemostasis: a 5-year overview. J Thromb Haemost. 2007;5:604–606.

[48] Voves C, Wuillemin WA, Zeerleder S. International Society on Thrombosis and Haemostasis score for overt disseminated intravascular coagulation predicts organ dysfunction and fatality in sepsis patients. Blood Coagul Fibrinolysis. 2006;17:445–451.

[49] Adam SS, Key NS, Greenberg CS. D-dimer antigen: current concepts and future prospects. Blood. 2009;113:2878–2887. DOI: 10.1182/blood-2008-06-165845.

[50] Wells PS, Anderson DR, Rodger M, Forgie M, Kearon C, Dreyer J, Kovacs G, Mitchell M, Lewandowski B, Kovacs MJ. Evaluation of D-dimer in the diagnosis of suspected deep-vein thrombosis. N Engl J Med. 2003;349:1227–1235.

[51] Schellong SM. Diagnosis of recurrent deep vein thrombosis. Hamostaseologie. 2013;33:195–200. DOI: 10.5482/HAMO-13-06-0029.

[52] van der Graaf F, van den Borne H, van der Kolk M, de Wild PJ, Janssen GW, van Uum SH. Exclusion of deep venous thrombosis with D-dimer testing – comparison of 13 D-dimer methods in 99 outpatients suspected of deep venous thrombosis using venography as reference standard. Thromb Haemost. 2000;83:191–198.

[53] Ghozlan MF, Osman AA, Mahmoud HM, Eissa DG. Comprehensive study on laboratory biomarkers for prediction and diagnosis of deep venous thrombosis. Blood Coagul Fibrinolysis. 2015;26:255–260. DOI: 10.1097/MBC.0000000000000164.

[54] Konstantinides S, Torbicki A. Management of venous thrombo-embolism: an update. Eur Heart J. 2014;35:2855–2863. DOI: 10.1093/eurheartj/ehu243.

[55] Xu J, Zhao J, Evan G, Xiao C, Cheng Y, Xiao J. Circulating microRNAs: novel biomarkers for cardiovascular diseases. J Mol Med (Berl). 2012;90:865–875. DOI: 10.1007/s00109-011-0840-5.

[56] Xu J, Lupu F, Esmon CT. Inflammation, innate immunity and blood coagulation. Hamostaseologie. 2010;30:5–6, 8–9.

[57] Morange PE, Tregouet DA. Lessons from genome-wide association studies in venous thrombosis. J Thromb Haemost. 2011;9:258–264. DOI: 10.1111/j.1538-7836.2011.04311.x.

[58] Zöller B, Li X, Sundquist J, Sundquist K. Familial transmission of venous thromboembolism: a cohort study of 80 214 Swedish adoptees linked to their biological and adoptive parents. Circ Cardiovasc Genet. 2014;7:296–303. DOI: 10.1161/CIRCGENETICS.113.000341.

[59] Vandy FC, Stabler C, Eliassen AM, Hawley AE, Guire KE, Myers DD, Henke PK, Wakefield TW. Soluble P-selectin for the diagnosis of lower extremity deep venous thrombosis. J Vasc Surg Venous Lymphat Disord. 2013;1:117–125.

[60] Hou H, Ge Z, Ying P, Dai J, Shi D, Xu Z, Chen D, Jiang, Q. Biomarkers of deep venous thrombosis. J Thromb Thrombolysis. 2012;34:335–346.

[61] Hoffman M. Remodeling the blood coagulation cascade. J Thromb Thrombolysis. 2003;16:17–20.

[62] Smith SA. The cell-based model of coagulation. J Vet Emer Crit Care (San Antonio). 2009;19:3–10. DOI: 10.1111/j.1476-4431.2009.00389.x.

[63] Sandset PM, Bends B, Hancen JB. Physiological function of tissue factor pathway inhibitor and interaction with heparins. Haemostasis. 2000;30:48–56.

[64] Hemker H, Giesen P, Al Dieri R, Regnault V, de Smed E, Wagenvoord R, Lecompte T, Béguin S. The calibrated automated thrombogramm (CAT): a universal routine test for hyper- and hypocoagulability. Pathophysiol Haemost Thromb. 2002;32:249–253.

[65] Hemker H, Giesen P, Al Dieri R, Regnault V, de Smedt E, Wagenvoord R, Lecompte T, Béguin S. Calibrated automated thrombin generation measurement in clotting plasma. Pathophysiol Haemost Thromb. 2003;33:4–15.

[66] McLean KC, Bernstein IM, Brummel-Ziedins K. Tissue factor dependent thrombin generation across pregnancy. Am J Obstet Gynecol. 2012;207:135e1–135e6. DOI: 10.1016/j.ajog.2012.05.027.

[67] Segers O, van Oerle Rv, ten Cate Ht, Rosing J, Castoldi E. Thrombin generation as an intermediate phenotype for venous thrombosis. Thromb Haemost. 2010;103:114–122. DOI: 10.1160/TH09-06-0356.

[68] van Veen JJ, Gatt A, Makris M. Thrombin generation testing in routine clinical practice: are we there yet? Br J Haematol. 2008;142:889–903. DOI: 10.1111/j.1365-2141.2008.07267.x.

[69] Momot A, Lydina I, Tsyvkina L, Borisova O, Serduk G. The Means of Progress in Improving the Results of in vitro Fertilization Based on the Identification and Correction of the Pathology of Hemostasis. In: Darwish AMM, editor. Enhancing Success of Assisted Reproduction. Rijeka, Croatia: InTech – Open Access Publisher; 2012. pp. 77–116. DOI: dx.doi.org/10.5772/3308

[70] Panteleev MA, Dashkevich NM, Ataullakhanov FI. Hemostasis and thrombosis beyond biochemistry: roles of geometry, flow and diffusion. Thromb Res. 2015;136:699–711. DOI: 10.1016/j.thromres.2015.07.025.

[71] Tarandovskiy ID, Balandina AN, Kopylov KG, Konyashina NI, Kumskova MA, Panteleev MA, Ataullakhanov FI. Investigation of the phenotype heterogeneity in severe hemophilia A using thromboelastography, thrombin generation, and thrombodynamics. Thromb Res. 2013;131:e274–e280. DOI: 10.1016/j.thromres.2013.04.004.

[72] Parunov LA, Soshitova NP, Fadeeva OA, Balandina AN, Kopylov KG, Kumskova MA, Gilbert JC, Schaub RG, McGinness KE, Ataullakhanov FI, Panteleev MA. Drug-drug interaction of the anti-TFPI aptamer BAX499 and factor VIII: studies of spatial dynamics of fibrin clot formation in hemophilia A. Thromb Res. 2014;133:112–119. DOI: 10.1016/j.thromres.2013.10.036.

[73] Gribkova IV, Spiridonova VA, Gorbatenko AS, Denisov SS, Ataullakhanov FI, Sinauridze EI. Thrombin inhibitors based on single-stranded DNA aptamers. Blood Coagul Fibrinolysis. 2014;25:39–45. DOI: 10.1097/MBC.0b013e32836577f3.

[74] Lindahl TL, Wallstedt M, Gustafsson KM, Persson E, Hillarp A. More efficient reversal of dabigatran inhibition of coagulation by activated prothrombin complex concentrates or recombinant factor VIIa than by four-factor prothrombin complex concentrate. Thromb Res. 2015;135:544–547. DOI: 10.1016/j.thromres.2014.12.019.

[75] Sinauridze EI, Kireev DA, Popenko NY, Pichugin AV, Panteleev MA, Krymskaya OV, Ataullakhanov FI. Platelet microparticle membranes have 50- to 100-fold higher specific procoagulant activity than activated platelets. Thromb Haemost. 2007;97:425–434.

[76] Soshitova NP, Karamzin SS, Balandina AN, Fadeeva OA, Kretchetova AV, Galstian GM, Panteleev MA, Ataullakhanov FI. Predicting prothrombotic tendencies in sepsis using spatial clot growth dynamics. Blood Coagul Fibrinolysis. 2012;23:498–507. DOI: 10.1097/MBC.0b013e328352e90e.

[77] Dashkevich NM, Ovanesov MV, Balandina AN, Karamzin SS, Shestakov PI, Soshitova NP, Tokarev AA, Panteleev MA, Ataullakhanov FI. Thrombin activity propagates in space during blood coagulation as an excitation wave. Biophys J. 2012;103:2233–2240. DOI: 10.1016/j.bpj.2012.10.011.

[78] Ataullakhanov FI, Dashkevich NM, Negrier C, Panteleev MA. Factor XI and traveling waves: the key to understanding coagulation in hemophilia? Expert Rev Hematol. 2013; 6:111–113. DOI: 10.1586/ehm.13.12.

Chapter 4

Management of Anticoagulation Around Cardiac Implantable Electronic Device Surgery

Roberto T. Sant´Anna, Tiago Luiz L. Leirira,
Pedro T. Sant´Anna and Gustavo G. Lima

Additional information is available at the end of the chapter

http://dx.doi.org/10.5772/64684

Abstract

The number of patients requiring cardiovascular implantable electronic device (CIED, e.g., pacemaker and defibrillator) surgery is increasing rapidly and at least a quarter of them are using chronic oral anticoagulation (OAC). Recently, the traditional approach of withholding anticoagulation and using heparin bridging has been challenged by studies showing safety of performing CIED surgery under anticoagulation with vitamin K antagonists. Bridging with heparin is associated with incremental healthcare costs, prolonged hospital admission, and also with an augmented relative risk of pocket hematoma. The risk of embolic events seems to be low and similar with the use of two strategies (heparin bridging and continuous warfarin). Experience with novel oral anticoagulants is limited. Few studies suggest that withholding 48–72 hours before surgery and performing the procedure under anticoagulation are safe alternatives. However, larger randomized clinical trials are needed before definitive conclusions. In this chapter, we review the management of anticoagulation around cardiac implantable electronic device surgery under new conditions.

Keywords: cardiac resynchronization therapy, implantable cardiac defibrillator, uninterrupted warfarin

1. Introduction

Each year, around 1.25 million pacemakers and 410,000 implantable cardioverter defibrillators (ICDs) are implanted worldwide. It is estimated that 25–35% of patients undergoing cardiac implantable electronic device (CIED) surgery receive long-term oral anticoagulation (OAC).

Many patients are also receiving oral antiplatelet therapy for primary or secondary cardiovascular events [1] and are exposed to an increased risk of bleeding during the perioperative period.

Pocket hematoma formation is the most common complication of CIED implantation [2]. Although benign in most cases, it can have serious consequences, such as prolongation of hospitalization, need for further surgery, and an increased risk of infection.

The periprocedural management of OAC poses a challenge, particularly in patients with moderate or higher risk (>5%/y) of arterial thromboembolic events (ATEs). Subtherapeutic anticoagulation exposes patients with atrial fibrillation (AF) to potential thromboembolic complications, with a calculated daily risk ranging from 0.01 to 0.05% [3]. Heparin is expected to reduce venous and arterial thromboembolism by 66–80% [4], but is associated with an increased risk of pocket hematoma.

Conversely, subtherapeutic anticoagulation exposes patients with AF to potential thromboembolic complications, with a calculated daily risk ranging from 0.01 to 0.05% [3]. This dilemma led some centers to perform this type of procedure without interrupting the OAC in patients deemed to be at a high risk for thromboembolic events.

2. Strategies for management of anticoagulation around CIED surgery

There are three perioperative anticoagulation strategies that can be employed:

1. Uninterrupted warfarin.

2. Withholding warfarin without bridging.

3. Withholding warfarin with perioperative bridging using heparin.

Theoretically, each strategy has its own advantages and limitations. The traditional strategy is to withhold warfarin with perioperative bridging using heparin in high-risk patients. This approach was linked to potential complications: a high risk of hematoma (between 17 and 31%), increased duration and costs of hospital stays, and increased risk of reoperation [5].

In a meta-analysis, we compared uninterrupted warfarin versus bridging using heparin. Maintenance of OAC, when compared to heparin bridge with unfractionated heparin or enoxaparin, had a lower risk of perioperative bleeding (OR = 0.25, 95% CI 0.17–0.36, $P < 0.00001$) (**Figure 1**). The risk of ATE was very low in our study, with only three events occurring in the group that received uninterrupted warfarin and one event in the group that received heparin bridging (OR = 1.86; 95% CI, 0.29–12.17; $P = 0.57$) [6].

Particularly, in the BRUISE study, thromboembolic events occurred in patients who were under OAC, but with INRs below the therapeutic range at the time of the event. Therefore, risk is probably more related to the adequacy of the anticoagulation control rather than the strategy applied.

Importantly, device pocket hematomas can necessitate prolonged cessation of anticoagulation with the attendant risk of ATE [6, 7]; they can significantly increase the duration and cost of hospitalization; and sometimes reoperation is required. Uslan et al. [8] have also highlighted the strong link between pocket hematoma and reintervention, the latter is an independent predictor of ICD infections.

Proietti et al. [9] found similar results in a meta-analysis with similar design that included 15 studies. Heparin bridging was associated with an increased risk of bleeding (OR = 4.47; 95% CI, 3.216.23; $P < 0.00001$), and prolonged hospital stay (9.13 ± 1.9 days vs. 5.11 ± 1.39 days; $P < 0.00001$). Adding heparin decreased the risk of ATE when compared with no anticoagulation (0.50% vs. 1.07%, $P = 0.02$), but there was no difference when heparin was compared with continuous OAC ($P = 0.83$). Results from this study discourage adoption of a strategy of OAC suspension with no heparin bridging.

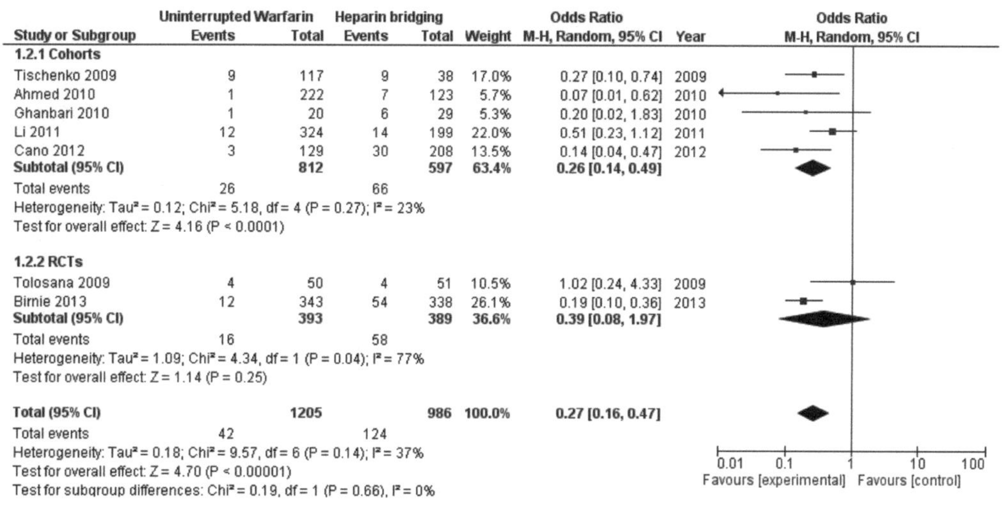

Figure 1. Risk of pocket hematoma in patients with oral anticoagulation continuation versus heparin bridging therapy, according to study design. Random effect model.

The BRIDGE study was a large randomized trial that compared bridging with low-molecular-weight heparin or placebo in patients anticoagulated with warfarin undergoing different types of surgeries [10]. Warfarin treatment was stopped 5 days before the procedure and was resumed within 24 hours after the procedure. During these periods, patients received low-molecular-weight heparin or placebo. Both groups had a similar low risk of ATE (0.4% in the no-bridging group and 0.3% in the bridging group). The incidence of major bleeding, however, was lower in the no-bridging group (relative risk, 0.41; 95% CI, 0.20–0.78; $P = 0.005$ for superiority).

This study included patients with low- to moderate-risk ATE—with a mean CHADS2 score of 2.3 and no mechanical heart valves. Studies during the perioperative period of CIED surgery included patients with moderate- to high-risk ATE. Also, CIED surgery represents a different scenario in which bleeding rarely is life threatening and is simple to diagnose. Therefore, we do not believe that results from BRIDGE should be applied to CIED surgery with the possible exception of patients with low risk of ATE.

The increased risk of bleeding related to heparin bridging has multiple causes. Feng et al. [11] hypothesize that the variations on the accuracy of monitoring of warfarin compared with heparin can partially explain differences in the observed risk of bleeding. Activated partial thromboplastin time (APTT) levels of 1.5–2.5 time control do not correlate well with the intensity of anticoagulation and have not been validated by randomized studies [12]. Moreover, heparin has antiplatelet effects that may last longer than the measurable effect of heparin and APTT [13]. Meanwhile, the evidence to maintain a therapeutic INR during the procedure is based on more consistent data of cohorts and randomized trials [14, 15]. Performing surgery under anticoagulation can facilitate the detection of small bleedings during the procedure [16]. This allows surgeons to make the necessary interventions at the time of the procedure and potentially reduce the risk of hematoma in the postoperative period. This phenomenon has been referred to as an "anticoagulation stress test."

Figure 2 shows a simplified guide for management of patients using OAC with vitamin K antagonists and requiring CIED surgery.

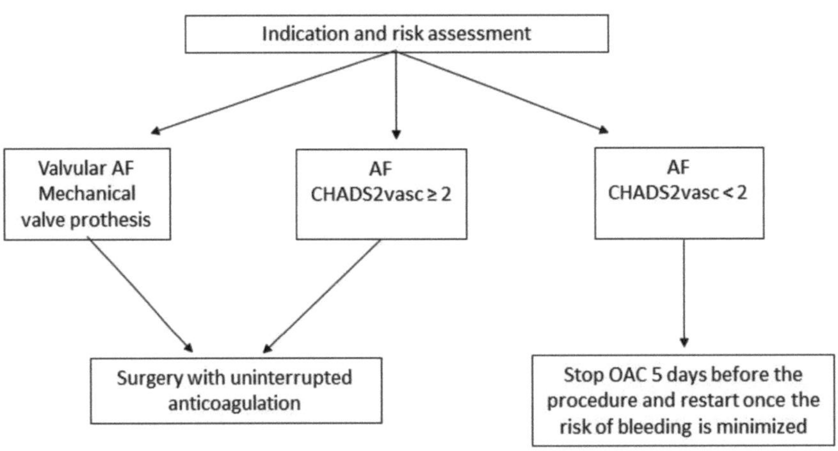

Figure 2. Guide for management of patients using OAC with vitamin K antagonists and requiring CIED surgery.

2.1. Role of novel anticoagulants

The use of novel anticoagulants (NOACs) has increased dramatically since its introduction with about 1/3 of patients with AF using them for stroke prophylaxis [17]. They represent a safe and efficacious alternative to warfarin. However, unlike warfarin, NOACs have a predictable dose-response curve. When prescribing these drugs, there is no need to monitor the INR levels to achieve therapeutic doses.

All NOACs are at least noninferior to warfarin in terms of efficacy for prevention of stroke in patients with nonvalvular AF [18–20]. In the same population, they are also at least as safe as warfarin in terms of major bleeding. NOACs are also at least as effective and as safe as warfarin for the treatment of venous thromboembolism [21, 22]. In patients with mechanical heart valves, dabigatran was inferior to warfarin in terms of stroke prevention and bleeding risk [23]; therefore, the use of NOAC was contraindicated in this population.

However, recommendations for periprocedural use of NOAC are not well established as they pose particular challenges:

1. Number of agents available on the market—dabigatran, rivaroxaban, apixaban, and edoxaban—each one with a unique pharmacokinetic profile.

2. Unavailability of an efficacious and widespread antidote in the case of urgent need to reverse anticoagulation.

3. Unavailability of a reliable laboratory test to measure the anticoagulation effect.

Some authors recommend that in patients with an annual risk of ATE (>5%), NOAC could be resumed 24 hours after surgery. In patients with a lower risk of ATE (<5%), it would seem reasonable to wait for >48 hours after surgery [24, 25].

Randomized trials like the planned BRUISE CONTROL-2 trial, which will compare continued vs. interrupted novel oral anticoagulant (dabigatran, rivaroxaban, or apixaban) at the time of device surgery [23], will bring more definitive answers.

In cases of clinical significant bleeding and need of urgent reversal of anticoagulation, several strategies have been studied and proposed in this setting. Mar et al. [26] suggest that if criteria for activated charcoal or hemodialysis use are not met, the use of four-factor prothrombin complex concentrate (25 U/kg, maximum dose of 2500 U) may be attempted to reverse dabigatran, as well as rivaroxaban and apixaban. Recently, a novel recombinant human factor Xa, andexanet alfa (AnXa), that binds with high affinity to apixaban and rivaroxaban has showed promising results in phase 3 studies [27].

Until more conclusive results are published, we recommend withholding NOAC four half-lives before elective procedures and restart the drug as soon as the risk of bleeding is minimized.

2.2. Cost-effectiveness

Bridging therapy is associated with increased costs due to increased need for hospitalization and the high price of LMWH [27]. In the BRUISE CONTROL STUDY, the overall cost of continued warfarin therapy was dramatically lower than heparin bridging therapy, primarily due to lower costs for medication and hospitalizations [28]. From the perspective of the Canadian healthcare system, continued warfarin therapy, when compared with heparin bridging, showed a cost saving of $1800 per patient.

2.3. Antithrombotic therapy in patients undergoing cardiac rhythm device implantation

Optimal management of antiplatelet therapy (AT) around CIED implantation is also challenging. Medications used as AT (e.g., aspirin and clopidogrel) have long half-lives and no efficient antidote; therefore, planning is essential to minimize the risk of bleeding while keeping a low risk of thrombotic complication.

Tompkins et al. reported that dual antiplatelet therapy in patients undergoing pacemaker implantation significantly increased frequency and severity of hemorrhagic complications, compared with the use of aspirin alone [29]. Other authors found no increased risk of bleeding complication in patients receiving clopidogrel or DAPT [30, 31].

ACC/AHA guidelines support continuing low-dose aspirin monotherapy for noncardiac surgical procedures, noting only a small increase in procedure-related bleeding (relative risk 1.5). Management of dual AT or clopidogrel use is still a matter of debate. Yang et al. performed a meta-analysis to evaluate the effects of different antiplatelet combinations in patients undergoing CIED surgery [1]. Dual antiplatelet therapy increased the risk of bleeding largely during CIED implantations compared with control group (OR = 6.84, 95% CI 4.16–11.25, $P < 0.00001$). Single antiplatelet therapy did not increase the risk of bleeding during CIED implantations (OR = 1.52, 95% CI 0.93–2.46, $P = 0.09$). Single antiplatelet therapy with clopidogrel increases the risk of hemorrhage when compared with aspirin (OR = 2.91, 95% CI 1.27–6.69, $P = 0.01$).

Abbreviations

AF	atrial fibrillation
ATE	arterial thromboembolic events
APTT	activated partial thromboplastin time
CIED	cardiac implantable electronic device
OAC	oral anticoagulation
NOAC	novel anticoagulant

Author details

Roberto T. Sant´Anna*, Tiago Luiz L. Leirira, Pedro T. Sant´Anna and Gustavo G. Lima

*Address all correspondence to: robertotofani@gmail.com

Instituto de Cardiologia, Fundação Universitária de Cardiologia, Porto Alegre, Brazil

http://dx.doi.org/10.5772/64684

References

[1] Yang X, Wang Z, Zhang Y, et al. The safety and efficacy of antithrombotic therapy in patients undergoing cardiac rhythm device implantation: a meta-analysis. Europace 2015; 17:1076–1084.

[2] Wiegand UKH, LeJeune D, Boguschewski F, Bonnemeier H, Eberhardt F, Bode HSF. Pocket hematoma after pacemaker or implantable cardioverter defibrillator surgery. Chest 2004; 126:1177.

[3] Vanleeuwen Y, Rosendaal FR, Cannegieter SC. Prediction of hemorrhagic and thrombotic events in patients with mechanical heart valve prostheses treated with oral anticoagulants. J Thromb Haemost 2008; 6:451–456.

[4] Kearon C, Hirsh J. Management of anticoagulation before and after elective surgery. N Engl J Med 1997; 336:1506–1515.

[5] Robinson M, Healey JS, Eikelboom J, et al. Postoperative low-molecular weight heparin bridging is associated with an increase in wound hematoma following surgery for pacemakers and implantable defibrillators. Pacing Clin Electrophysiol 2009; 32:378–382.

[6] Sant'anna RT, Leiria TL, Nascimento T, et al. Meta-analysis of continuous oral anticoagulants versus heparin bridging in patients undergoing CIED surgery: reappraisal after the BRUISE study. PACE 2015; 38:417–423.

[7] Romeyer-Bouchard C, Da Costa A, et al. Prevalence and risk factors related to infections of cardiac resynchronization therapy devices. Eur Heart J 2010; 31:203–210.

[8] Uslan DZ, Gleva MJ, Warren DK, et al. Cardiovascular implantable electronic device replacement infections and prevention: results from the REPLACE Registry. Pacing Clin Electrophysiol 2012; 35:81–87.

[9] Proietti R, Porto I, Levi M, et al. Risk of pocket hematoma in patients on chronic anticoagulation with warfarin undergoing electrophysiological device implantation: a comparison of different peri-operative management strategies. Eur Rev Med Pharmacol Sci 2015; 19:1461–1479.

[10] Douketis JD, Spyropoulos AC, Kaatz S, et al. Perioperative bridging anticoagulation in patients with atrial fibrillation. N Engl J Med 2015; 373:823–833.

[11] Feng L, Li Y, Li J, et al. Oral anticoagulation continuation (compared with heparin bridging therapy among high risk patients undergoing implantation of cardiac rhythm devices: a meta-analysis. Thromb Haemost 2012; 108:1124–1131.

[12] Basu D, Gallus A, Hirsh J, et al. A prospective study of the value of monitoring heparin treatment with the activated partial thromboplastin time. N Engl J Med 1972; 287:324–327.

[13] Carr ME Jr, Carr SL. At high heparin concentrations, protamine concentrations which reverse heparin anticoagulant effects are insufficient to reverse heparin anti-platelet effects. Thromb Res 1994; 15:617–630.

[14] Johnston M, Harrison L, Moffat K, et al. Reliability of the international normalized ratio for monitoring the induction phase of warfarin: comparison with the prothrombin time ratio. J Lab Clin Med 1996; 128:214–217.

[15] van den Besselaar AM, Chantarangkul V, et al. Thromboplastin standards. Biologicals 2010; 38:430–436.

[16] Birnie DH, Healey JS, Wells GA, et al. Pacemaker or defibrillator surgery without interruption of anticoagulation. N Engl J Med 2013; 368:2084–2093.

[17] Lauffenburger JC, Farley JF, Gehi AK, et al. Factors driving anticoagulant selection in patients with atrial fibrillation in the United States. Am J Cardiol. 2015; 115:1095–1101.

[18] Connolly SJ, Ezekowitz MD, Yusuf S, et al. Dabigatran versus warfarin in patients with atrial fibrillation. N Engl J Med 2009; 361:1139–1151.

[19] Granger CB, Alexander JH, McMurray JJ, et al. Apixaban versus warfarin in patients with atrial fibrillation. N Engl J Med 2011; 365:981–992.

[20] Patel MR, Mahaffey KW, Garg J, et al. Rivaroxaban versus warfarin in nonvalvular atrial fibrillation. N Engl J Med 2011; 365:883–891.

[21] Agnelli G, Buller HR, Cohen A, et al. Oral apixaban for the treatment of acute venous thromboembolism. N Engl J Med 2014; 369:799–808.

[22] Bauersachs R, Berkowitz SD, Brenner B, et al. Oral rivaroxaban for symptomatic venous thromboembolism. N Engl J Med 2010; 363:2499–2510.

[23] Eikelboom JW, Connolly SJ, Brueckmann M, et al. Dabigatran versus warfarin in patients with mechanical heart valves. N Engl J Med 2013; 369:1206–1214.

[24] Birnie DH, Healey JS, Essebag V. Management of anticoagulation aroundpacemaker and defibrillator surgery. Circulation 2014; 129:2062–2065.

[25] Essebag V, Healey JS, Ayala-Paredes F, et al. Strategy of continued vs. interrupted novel oral anticoagulant at time of device surgery in patients with moderate to high risk of arterial thromboembolic events: The BRUISE CONTROL-2 trial. Am Heart Journal 2016; 173:102–107.

[26] Gold M, Crowther M, Levy G, et al. Annexatm-R: a Phase 3 randomized, double-blind, placebo-controlled trial, demonstrating reversal of rivaroxaban-induced anticoagulation in older subjects by andexanet alfa (Prt064445), a universal antidote for factor Xa (Fxa) inhibitors. J Am Coll Cardiol 2015; 65:A23.

http://dx.doi.org/10.5772/64684

[27] Spyropoulos AC, Jenkins P, Bornikova L. A disease management protocol for outpatient perioperative bridge therapy with enoxaparin in patients requiring temporary interruption of long-term oral anticoagulation. Pharmacotherapy 2004; 24:649–658.

[28] Coyle D, Coyle K, Essebag V, et al. Cost effectiveness of continued-warfarin versus heparin-bridging therapy during pacemaker and defibrillator surgery. J Am Coll Cardiol 2015; 65:957–959.

[29] Tompkins C, Cheng A, Dalal D, et al. Dual antiplatelet therapy and heparin "bridging" significantly increase the risk of bleeding complications after pacemaker or implantable cardioverter-defibrillator device implantation. J Am Coll Cardiol 2010; 55:2376–2382.

[30] Ozcan KS, Osmonov D, Yildirim E, et al. Hematoma complicating permanent pacemaker implantation: the role of periprocedural antiplatelet or anticoagulant therapy. J Cardiol 2013; 62:127–130.

[31] Przybylski A, Derejko P, Kwasniewski W, et al. Bleeding complications after pacemaker or cardioverter defibrillator implantation in patients receiving dual antiplatelet therapy: results of a prospective, two-center registry. Neth Heart J 2010; 18:230–235.

Chapter 5

Prothrombin Complex Concentrate, a General Antidote for Oral Anticoagulation

Herm Jan M. Brinkman

Additional information is available at the end of the chapter

http://dx.doi.org/10.5772/64304

Abstract

Prothrombin complex concentrate (PCC) is used for the rapid reversal of vitamin K antagonist (VKA) anticoagulation. PCC is also applicable in situations requiring rapid reversal of anticoagulation by non-vitamin K antagonist direct thrombin and factor Xa inhibitor oral anticoagulants (NOACs), thereby making PCC a general antidote for oral anticoagulation. In this chapter, the composition of different PCC brands is reviewed and a negative effect of heparin supplement in some products is recognized. Mode of action of anticoagulation reversal by PCC is explained. Dosage and clinical efficacy, two closely related issues, are discussed and based on reviewed data recommendations are given that may prohibit too low PCC dosing, especially in NOAC anticoagulation. Use of unsuitable laboratory assays has raised needless controversy as to the applicability of PCC to reverse anticoagulation by NOACs, in particular dabigatran. In this chapter, various laboratory assays are evaluated for their applicability in monitoring reversal of anticoagulation.

Keywords: vitamin K antagonists, rivaroxaban, dabigatran, direct oral anticoagulants, prothrombin complex concentrate

1. Introduction

Fluidity of circulating blood is maintained by a delicate balance between procoagulant and anticoagulant processes. A complex mechanism involving the vessel wall, platelets, and proteins in plasma (clotting factors) safeguards a normal blood flow by the formation of a blood clot at sites of vessel damage [1–3]. Upon vessel damage, platelets rapidly deposit at the site of vascular injury. Tissue factor that is normally sequestered from circulating blood, now triggers a cascade of biochemical reactions among coagulation proteins resulting in the formation of thrombin, the enzyme that converts fibrinogen into fibrin (**Figure 1**). A blood clot consists of a mesh of fibrin threads, aggregated platelets, leukocytes, and erythrocytes. Thrombosis is the formation of blood clots or thrombi inside the blood vessel or on surgical implants. Clots can cause partial or complete blockade of the blood flow. A serious complication that can arise from thrombosis is embolism, which refers to a condition in which a portion of the blood clot breaks loose and travels in the bloodstream. Emboli can obstruct vessels in other parts of the body. Vessel occlusion can lead to severe tissue damage. Thrombosis is clearly one of the most common causes of death. A measure to prevent thrombosis is the use of anticoagulant drugs [4]. Classic oral anticoagulant drugs, the vitamin K antago-

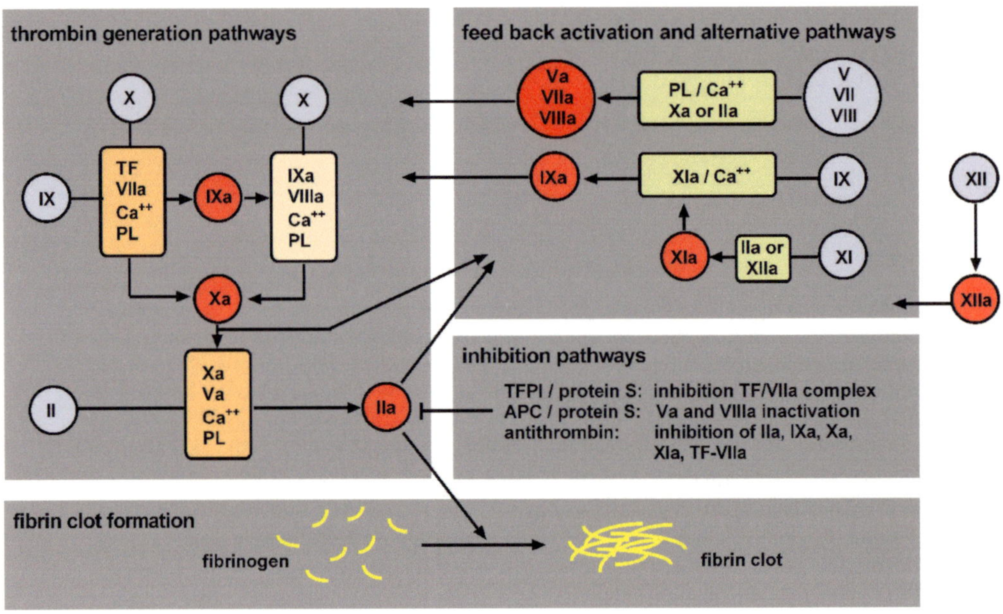

Figure 1. Pathways involved in thrombin generation and fibrin clot formation. Extrinsic coagulation starts with the binding of factor VII and activated factor VII (VIIa) to tissue factor (TF) on the outer layer of the lipid membrane of perivascular cells exposed to blood upon vessel wall damage. Factor VIIa bound to TF is able to proteolytically activate the coagulation factors IX and X. Additional factor X activation occurs by activated factor IX (IXa) when assembled with its active cofactor factor VIIIa on a negatively charged phospholipid surface (PL), e.g. the surface of an activated blood platelet. Subsequently, factor Xa assembles on a PL surface with its active cofactor, factor Va, as such able to proteolytically activate prothrombin (II). Without the respective active cofactors Va and VIIIa, factor IXa and factor Xa display very poor enzymatic activity. Formation of thrombin (IIa) is accelerated by feedback activation of factor V and VIII as well as factor VII by initially formed small amounts of factor Xa and thrombin. Another feedback loop involves the activation of factor XI by thrombin that facilitates additional factor IX activation. Note that reactions that require PL are calcium-ion (Ca++) dependent. Intrinsic coagulation (contact activation) is triggered by the conversion of factor XII into its enzymatic active form (XIIa) that occurs on negatively charged polyphosphates such as RNA, DNA, and inorganic polyphosphate that are released during cell damage and infection. Intrinsic coagulation is not regarded as the physiological pathway. Thrombin generation is under control of several inhibitory pathways. Tissue factor pathway inhibitor (TFPI) blocks the TF/VIIa complex when assembled with factor Xa. Protein C, once activated (APC) by thrombin when bound to thrombomodulin on the vessel wall, proteolytically inactivates the cofactors Va and VIIIa. Both processes are enhanced in the presence of protein S. Antithrombin inactivates thrombin, factor IXa, Xa, XIa, as well as factor VIIa bound to TF. The anticoagulant function of antithrombin is significantly enhanced by heparin-like structures on the vessel wall.

nists (VKAs), inhibit the essential modification of newly synthesized vitamin K-dependent coagulation factors in the liver. Other, more recently developed non-vitamin K antagonist oral anticoagulants (NOACs) only target specific clotting factors in their enzymatic active configuration. A significant side effect of (oral) anticoagulation therapy is the increased risk of bleeding [5–7]. Rapid reversal of anticoagulation might be required in anticoagulated patients presenting with major bleeding or requiring urgent surgery or invasive intervention.

To date, fresh frozen plasma (FFP) is still being used for the treatment of hemorrhages associated with the use of oral VKA anticoagulant drugs that interfere in the synthesis of vitamin K-dependent clotting factors in the liver. This is despite the availability of much more effective prothrombin complex concentrate or PCC [8–12]. Major disadvantages associated with FFP therapy include the risk of transfusion-related acute lung injury (TRALI), the need to consider blood group compatibility, and the large volume of intravenously administered plasma needed to stop bleeding episodes with concomitant risk of systemic volume overload [13]. In the late 1950s and much of the 1960s, FFP was the mainstay of treatment of bleeding associated with coagulation factor deficiencies like hemophilia A (congenital factor VIII deficiency) and hemophilia B (congenital factor IX deficiency). Hemophilia treatment improved in the late 1960s by the introduction of partly purified, human plasma-derived concentrates of either factor VIII or factor IX. Factor IX belongs to the group of vitamin K-dependent proteins, including, among others, the procoagulant factors II (prothrombin), VII, IX, and X. Due to the presence of the other vitamin K-dependent coagulation factors in partly purified factor IX concentrates, its use was also recognized for the treatment of congenital factor VII and factor X deficiencies, as well as for acquired deficiencies in vitamin K-dependent coagulation factors due to liver disease [14]. And last but not least, partly purified factor IX concentrates appeared extremely useful in rapid reversal of anticoagulation by vitamin K antagonists like warfarin [15, 16]. Nowadays, partly purified factor IX concentrate is referred to as prothrombin complex concentrate (PCC). An old abbreviation still being used is PPSB (prothrombin, proconvertin, Stuart-Prower-factor, Christmas factor/Factor B).

2. Prothrombin complex concentrate and indications of its clinical use

2.1. Reversal of vitamin K antagonists

Three different types of PCCs are commercially available for clinical use (**Table 1**): four-factor (4F) PCC, three-factor (3F) PCC, and activated PCC. The functional procoagulant components in 4F-PCC are the vitamin K-dependent coagulation factors II (prothrombin), VII, IX, and X. Brand names, among others, are Beriplex® (Kcentra™ in the USA), Octaplex®, Prothromplex®, and Cofact®. 3F-PCC, in contrast to its 4F counterpart, does not contain significant levels of factor VII. Brand names include Profilnine® and Bebulin®. Activated PCC (Feiba®) contains the proenzymes prothrombin (factor II), factor IX, and factor X as in 3F-PCC and 4F-PCC, but in addition contains factor VII in its activated form (VIIa) (see **Figure 2**). Of these PCCs, 4F-PCC is approved as reversal agent for VKAs. In the US, approval is granted by the Food and Drug Administration (FDA) for urgent reversal of acquired coagulation factor

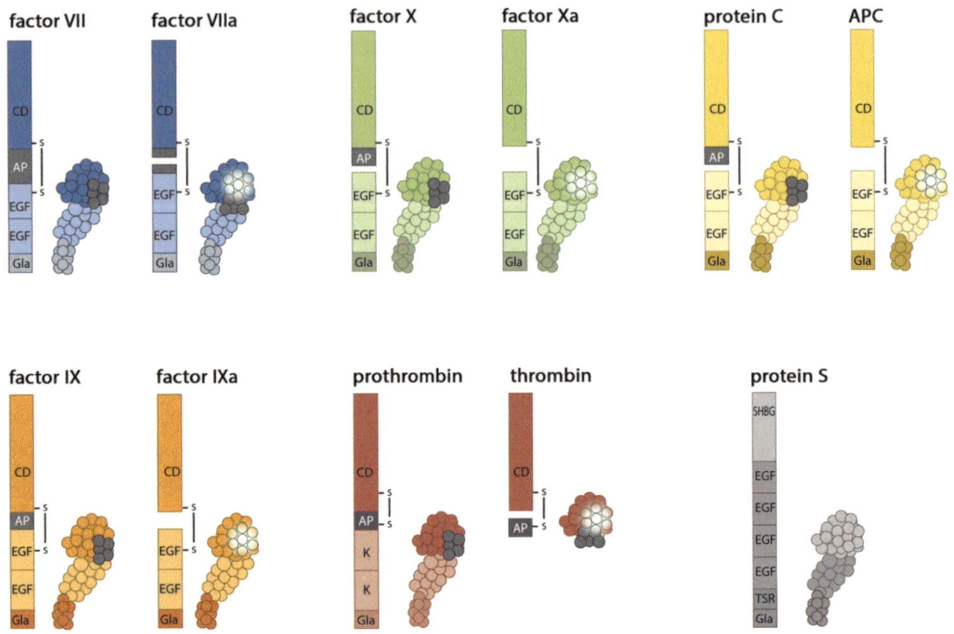

Figure 2. Vitamin K-dependent coagulation proteins. Vitamin K-dependent procoagulant factors (VII, IX, X, prothrombin) and vitamin K-dependent anticoagulant proteins (C and S) are depicted as bars illustrating their different domains as well as globular structures based on current knowledge of their three dimensional configuration [55–65]. Vitamin K-dependent clotting factors consist of a so-called Gla domain, one or more EGF or Kringle domains, and a catalytic domain (CD). Protein S does not contain a catalytic domain and instead contains a so-called SHBG domain. The Gla domain is essential for binding to negatively charged phospholipids, e.g. present in the outer layer of the membrane of activated platelets. The enzymatic activity of vitamin K-dependent clotting factors resides in the catalytic domain. In pro-enzymes, the site that is responsible for the proteolytic activity is masked. The active site becomes exposed upon proteolytic cleavage of the so-called activation peptide (AP). In factor VIIa and thrombin, the cleaved activation peptide remains attached. In factor IXa, factor Xa, and activated protein C, the activation peptide is cleaved out. Thrombin has lost its Kringle domains and its Gla domain and therefore is not able to bind to negatively charged phospholipids. Thrombin, in most cases, exerts its activity in solution and independent of a phospholipid membrane. Protein S does not contain an activation peptide and catalytic domain, and therefore cannot exhibit enzymatic activity.

deficiency induced by VKA therapy in patients with acute major bleeding only. In various countries outside the US, 4F-PCC is indicated for emergency as well as prophylactic reversal of VKA anticoagulation and for replacement therapy in patients with congenital or acquired factor deficiencies. Given their composition, 4F-PCCs may provide an off-label alternative for treatment of acute bleeds in patients with liver disease and in patients with trauma-induced coagulopathy [17]. 3F-PCC is approved in several countries including the US for hemophilia B treatment. Clinical studies indicate that 3F-PCC can also be used for the reversal of anticoagulation by vitamin K antagonists, albeit less effective than 4F-PCC [18–21]. Activated PCC is indicated in situations where a factor VIII or IX inhibitor bypassing procoagulant drug is required. Its off-label use as reversal agent for VKA-induced coagulopathy seems obvious because of its composition (presence of all procoagulant vitamin K-dependent factors, with factor VII in its activated form). The clinical usefulness of activated PCC in emergency reversal of vitamin K antagonists has been demonstrated in a limited number of clinical studies [10, 22].

Concentrate	Major functional component(s)	Indications*	Off-label use/remark
4F-PCC	Coagulation factors II, VII, IX, X	Treatment and perioperative prophylaxis of bleeding – in acquired deficiency of PCC factors, such as deficiency caused by treatment with vitamin K antagonists – in congenital deficiency of the vitamin K-dependent coagulation factors when purified specific coagulation factor products are not available	Treatment of trauma-induced coagulopathy Treatment of bleeds in patients with liver disease Reversal of anticoagulation by direct factor Xa and thrombin-inhibiting oral anticoagulants (evidence based on several bleeding models in animals and human volunteers; substantial clinical evidence is lacking)
3F-PCC	Coagulation factors II, IX, X	Prevention and control of bleeding in hemophilia B patients	Anticoagulant reversal agent – for vitamin K antagonists (4F-PCC is superior to 3F-PCC) – for direct oral thrombin and factor Xa inhibitors (evidence based on a few bleeding models in animals; substantial clinical evidence is lacking)
Activated-PCC	Coagulation factors II, IX, X, VII-activated form	Treatment and prophylaxis of bleeding in patients (hemophilia A and B as well as non-hemophiliacs) with inhibitors to factors VIII or IX	Anticoagulant reversal agent – for vitamin K antagonists (evidence based on a limited number of clinical studies) – for direct oral thrombin and factor Xa inhibitors (evidence based on bleeding models in animals; substantial clinical evidence is lacking)
Factor VIIa	Coagulation factor VII-activated form	Treatment and perioperative prophylaxis of bleeding – in hemophilia patients with acquired inhibitors to factors VIII or IX – in patients with congenital factor VII deficiency	Treatment of intracranial hemorrhage and control of bleeding in trauma and during surgery Anticoagulant reversal agent – for vitamin K antagonists (lacking substantial clinical evidence; may require co-administration of FFP or 3F-PCC) – for direct oral thrombin and factor Xa inhibitors (evidence based on bleeding models in animals; substantial clinical evidence is lacking)
Factor VIII	Coagulation factor VIII	Treatment and prophylaxis of bleeding in patients with hemophilia A	Not to be used as anticoagulant reversal agent
Factor IX	Coagulation factor IX	Treatment and prophylaxis of bleeding in patients with hemophilia B	Not to be used as anticoagulant reversal agent

*According to summary of product characteristics (SPC).

Table 1. Clotting factor concentrates; indications and off-label use.

In this context, we should also mention recombinant activated factor VII (VIIa) concentrate (NovoSeven®). This factor concentrate was originally developed for the treatment of bleeding in patients with hemophilia who developed antibodies to factor VIII. Off-label use of recombinant factor VIIa has been documented in a number of bleeding conditions including cardiovascular surgery, trauma, and intracranial hemorrhage [23]. Some case-control studies have suggested a beneficial effect of a factor VIIa concentrate in the treatment of VKA-associated bleeds [24–27]. Off-label use of recombinant factor VIIa as VKA antidote is usually in combination with FFP therapy. A recent report outlined the successful use of a combination of recombinant factor VIIa and 3F-PCC in the treatment of VKA-associated intracranial hemorrhage [28]. The idea behind the treatment of hemorrhages with recombinant factor VIIa is the delivery of a sufficient amount of already activated factor VII to exposed tissue factor at sites of vessel injury (**Figure 1**). In an alternative model, recombinant factor VIIa interacts with the GPIb-IX-V complex on platelets and this interaction enhances tissue factor-independent thrombin generation mediated by recombinant factor VIIa on the activated platelet surface [29]. When employing recombinant factor VIIa concentrate, one should keep in mind that sufficient plasma levels of other essential vitamin K-dependent coagulation factors are still needed (**Figure 1**). In VKA-anticoagulated subjects, levels of functional vitamin K-dependent clotting factors may be too low to support recombinant factor VIIa treatment in the absence of FFP or 3F-PCC. This notion is underscored by the absence of a significant correcting effect of recombinant factor VIIa concentrate in carefully controlled bleeding models in rats (tail injury), mice (tail injury), and human volunteers (punch biopsy) subjected to VKA anticoagulation [30–32]. Interestingly, correction of bleeding did occur in incomplete anticoagulated rats [30]. On the other hand, two studies reported recombinant factor VIIa to be effective in reducing VKA-associated experimental intracerebral hemorrhage in mice [33, 34]. Co-administration of FFP or 3F-PCC was omitted in all referred model studies. Thus, although data are inconclusive on this matter, effective emergency reversal of VKA anticoagulation by recombinant factor VIIa may require the co-administration of FFP or 3F-PCC.

2.2. Reversal of direct thrombin and factor Xa inhibitors

NOACs are the new generation oral anticoagulants that directly inhibit thrombin (factor IIa) or activated factor X (Xa). A treatment algorithm for NOAC-associated bleeds has been developed that includes the use of PCC [35]. Studies employing bleeding models in animals and healthy human volunteers have revealed that all PCCs as well as recombinant factor VIIa are potentially applicable in the treatment of NOAC-associated bleeds [36]. Most well studied is the reversal of NOAC anticoagulation by 4F-PCC, with seven out of eight studies showing partial to complete bleeding cessation in coagulopathy induced by direct factor Xa inhibitors (apixaban 2/2, edoxaban 2/2, rivaroxaban 3/4) and 5/6 in that induced by the direct thrombin inhibitor dabigatran [32, 37–49]. 3F-PCC was successfully explored in the reversal of dabigatran-induced hemorrhage in rat [48]. Activated PCC was shown to reduce dabigatran- as well as rivaroxaban-associated bleeds in various bleeding models [32, 45, 48, 50]. Results with factor VIIa concentrate were less conclusive, showing positive outcome in about half of the reported bleeding models [32, 43–49]. Several reasons may underlie the variability in study outcome, including the bleeding model used, plasma concentration of the NOAC

http://dx.doi.org/10.5772/64304

at the time of intervention, and the type and dosage of reversal agent administered. The composition of the PCC, that differs from brand to brand, may also be of influence. Case reports and clinical registries have described multiple interventions in the treatment of NOAC-associated emergency bleeds, including the use of 4F-PCC, activated PCC, and recombinant factor VIIa [51–54]. There is currently no strong clinical evidence (e.g. randomized controlled trials) to support the choice of one of the hemostatic agents.

3. What is in the vial?

3.1. Vitamin K-dependent coagulation proteins

PCC is a mixture of partly purified vitamin K-dependent coagulation proteins (**Figure 2**). PCCs are prepared from human plasma and are supplied as freeze-dried products. Dosage indicated on the label and package insert of 3F- and 4F-PCC is based on the factor IX content and is given in international activity units (IU) factor IX as assayed according the prescriptions in the European Pharmacopeia. In contrast, the potency of activated PCC (Feiba®) is expressed in arbitrary units defined as that amount able to shorten the clotting time of factor VIII inhibitor reference plasma to 50% of normal.

Some of the earlier PCCs available until the mid-1990s were associated with an increased risk of thrombosis [66]. Data published by Grundman et al. suggest that prothrombin overload caused by an imbalance of coagulation factors in PCC is the major thrombogenic trigger during PCC therapy [67]. An appropriate balance in the levels of coagulation factors may therefore have significant influence on the safety of PCC [68]. Most desirable are relative clotting factor quantities similar to that in plasma. In **Figure 3**, molar quantities of the different clotting factors

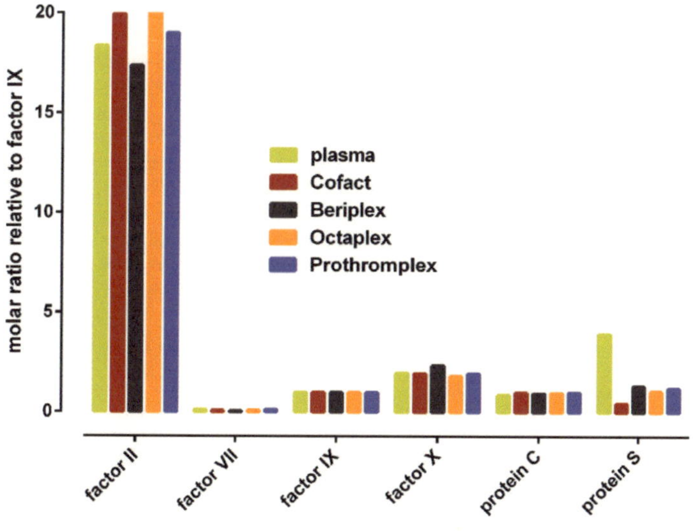

Figure 3. Vitamin K-dependent plasma proteins in plasma and in 4F-PCC. See legend **Table 2** for analytical details.

relative to factor IX are shown for some of the currently available PCCs. As can be appreciated, relative quantities of all procoagulant vitamin K-dependent clotting factors in PCC are almost identical to that in plasma. This is also true for the vitamin K-dependent coagulation inhibitor protein C. For protein S, however, levels are considerably lower than in plasma. Prothrombin is the most abundant vitamin K-dependent coagulation factor, while only trace amounts of factor VII are present in both plasma and PCC.

3.2. Other plasma protein constituents

PCCs not only contain vitamin K-dependent coagulation proteins. Mass spectrometric analysis revealed the presence of a variety of common plasma proteins such as fibrinogen, vitronectin, inter-alpha-trypsin inhibitor, complement, albumin, ceruloplasmin, C4b-binding protein, and apolipoprotein [69, 70]. The amount of co-purified plasma constituents may vary between the different PCC brands. Copper-containing ceruloplasmin is responsible for the bluish colour of some PCCs.

Biochemical characteristics		**PCC product**			
		Cofact	**Beriplex**	**Octaplex**	**Prothromplex**
Specific activity	IU factor IX/mg total protein	1.7 (1.1)	4.8 (3.3)	0.9 (1.0)	1.7 (1.5)
Vitamin K-dependent coagulation proteins	mg, % of total protein	22 (23)	59 (42)	12 (14)	24 (-)
Antithrombin	IU/IU factor IX	0.01 (0.01)	0.02 (0.02)	0.004 (0.003–0.004)	0.03 (0.03–0.06)
Heparin supplement	IU/IU factor IX	<0.01 (<0.01)	0.03 (0.02–0.03)	0.25 (0.15–0.88)	0.38 (0.15–0.72)
Thrombin generation	ETP, % of control plasma	217	162	71	18

From each product, a single lot was analyzed at Sanquin laboratories. Factor IX activity (clotting assay) was determined against the European Pharmacopoeia reference standard for factor IX concentrates. Prothrombin, factor VII, factor X, protein C, antithrombin (all chromogenic assays), and protein S (total antigen) were calculated against WHO calibrated normal plasma. IU was recalculated to mg based on reference plasma quantities as listed in the corresponding ISTH-SSC subcommittee communication [72]. Total protein was determined according to Bradford [71]. Heparin was determined against the 6th international standard for unfractionated heparin [73]. Thrombin generation (CAT method) in normal plasma supplemented with 1 IU/ml PCC was performed as described using a tissue factor concentration of 5 pM [73]. ETP values (extrinsic thrombin generation, area under the thrombin generation cure) are expressed as % of those obtained in normal plasma supplemented with saline instead of PCC. Content may vary from lot to lot. Data obtained are in good agreement with values from the literature, as can be appreciated from the data between parentheses that were taken directly from reports by Kalina et al., Sadeghi et al. and Grottke et al. or that were calculated from the reported values [74–76]. -, no literature data available.

Table 2. Biochemical characterization of 4F-PCC.

Specific activity is a measure of purity. Specific activity of 3F- and 4F-PCC is the amount of factor IX activity (in IU) over the total amount of all proteins (in mg) present in the product. Total protein is determined spectrophotometrically employing a protein dye and the levels are calculated using a calibration curve of an albumin solution with known protein content [71]. Specific activities of some currently available PCCs are listed in **Table 2**. Dissimilar specific activities of the different PCCs are indicative for differences in composition and purity. Specific activity based on factor IX coagulant activity, however, does not take into account therapeutic vitamin K-dependent coagulation factors other than factor IX. In **Table 2**, the sum of mg quantities of the factors II, VII, IX, X, protein C, and protein S in 4F-PCC is expressed as percentage of total protein. This calculation reveals a purity that varies between 12 and 59%.

3.3. Heparin and antithrombin supplement: its influence on PCCs procoagulant potential

In the early days of PCC utilization, clinicians were facing an increased incidence of thrombosis in PCC-treated patients [66]. To minimize thrombogenicity, heparin and antithrombin were advised as supplements in PCC [68]. With the inclusion of coagulation inhibitors and other manufacturing improvements and the implementation of thrombogenicity release tests, today's PCCs can be considered safer than earlier products [77]. The rationale behind heparin and antithrombin supplementation is to inactivate any activated coagulation factor in the final PCC product. Levels of heparin and antithrombin supplement, however, vary considerably between different PCC brands (**Table 2**). The ability of heparin and antithrombin supplement to inhibit any active coagulation factor in PCC can be demonstrated, e.g. by mixing PCC with active thrombin. The level of antithrombin appeared to have greater impact on thrombin inhibition than either heparin content or the ratio of antithrombin to heparin [74].

The presence of antithrombin and heparin supplement may have influence on the procoagulant potential of the PCC, i.e. the ability to reverse oral anticoagulation. A negative effect of anticoagulant supplement can be easily demonstrated in the so-called thrombin generation test. In this test, thrombin generation in a plasma sample is initiated by the addition of calcium-ions and a trigger of coagulation, usually tissue factor. A fluorogenic, thrombin-sensitive substrate is present in the incubation mixture, allowing to monitor in time the generation and subsequent inhibition of thrombin [78]. The area under the thrombin generation curve (endogenous thrombin potential, ETP), one of the parameters that can be derived from the curve, is frequently used as a measure for the amount of thrombin generated. When PCC is added to normal plasma, an increase in ETP is to be expected because of an increase in level of all essential coagulation factors. An increase in ETP can indeed be observed with Cofact® and to a lesser extent with Beriplex®, PCCs that contain no or little heparin (**Table 2**). Octaplex® and Prothromplex®, PCCs with a considerable amount of heparin supplement, show inhibition of coagulation with this test (**Table 2**). A correlation between ETP and the quantity of antithrombin supplement seems absent.

Several reports have pointed to a potential negative effect of heparin supplement on the procoagulant efficacy of PCC [73, 76, 79–81]; though all of these are in vitro studies, a clinical effect should not be ruled out. Let us envision a patient on rivaroxaban anticoagulation treated for an emergency bleed with the advised dose of PCC of 50 IU factor IX/kg body weight (bw), infused at a generally practiced flow rate of 2.5 IU factor IX/kg bw per min [82]. This means that, depending on the PCC administered (see **Table 2**), in total up to 36 IU heparin/kg bw at a rate of 1.8 IU heparin/kg bw per min (108 IU heparin/kg bw per h) is infused. Clinicians thus should be aware of the possibility that during PCC infusions and depending on the PCC brand administered, levels of co-administered heparin may be within the heparin therapeutic window [83]. PCC infusion, however, is temporary (±25 min for 50 IU/kg) and the half-life of heparin (30–60 min) is relatively short as compared to that of factor II (45–66 h), factor VII (4–7 h), factor IX (14–68 h) and factor X (24–41 h) [83, 84]. It is therefore to be expected that co-infused heparin may only transiently counteract the prohemostatic efficacy of administered clotting factor concentrate. Additional complicating aspect when treating emergency bleeds in patient on rivaroxaban or any other NOAC, is the fact that co-infused heparin supplement will enhance the anticoagulant effect of the NOAC (see **Figure 4** and reference [73]). Thus, an inhibitory effect of heparin during and shortly after infusion of heparin-containing PCC should be taken into account, especially when treating emergency bleeds associated with NOAC anticoagulation. PCC brands containing no or low heparin do not have this side effect.

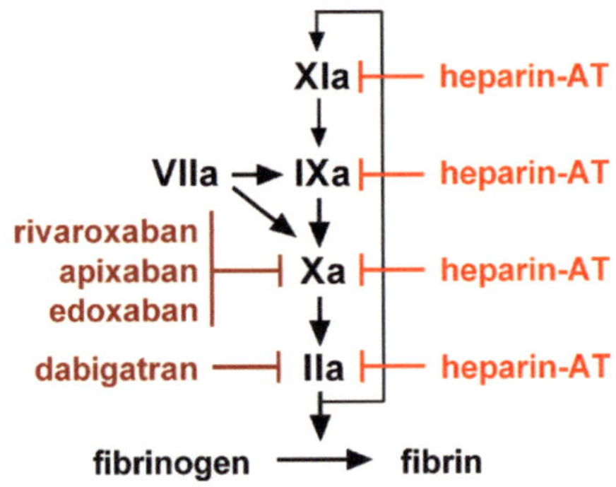

Figure 4. Heparin intensifies NOAC anticoagulation. Coagulation enzymes are inhibited by antithrombin (AT), a process significantly enhanced by heparin. Rivaroxaban, apixaban, and edoxaban are direct Xa inhibitors. Dabigatran is a direct thrombin inhibitor. Heparin supplement present in some PCCs and direct Xa and thrombin inhibitors (NOACs) act synergistically to depress coagulation [73]. It would therefore be more beneficial to treat emergency bleeds in NOAC-anticoagulated individuals with PCCs containing no or low dose heparin than with PCCs containing high dose heparin. (Coagulation cofactors are not depicted in this schematic representation.)

3.4. Activated coagulation factors and release tests

Release tests for manufactured PCC should comply with European Pharmacopoeia monographs [85]. Release tests, among others, include solubility, sterility, bacterial endotoxins, coagulation factor II, VII, IX, X, and activated coagulation factors. Heparin, if present in the PCC, must be neutralized when performing coagulation factor and activated coagulation factor release tests. Thrombin is measured by mixing prescribed volumes of PCC and fibrinogen solution. If thrombin is present, fibrin will be formed. PCC batches only pass this test if fibrin formation is absent in one test tube kept at 37°C for 6 h and in another tube kept at room temperature for 24 h. For comparison, coagulation occurs within 30 s in a reference tube containing a prescribed mixture of fibrinogen and thrombin instead of PCC. The absence of thrombin in currently available PCCs was recently confirmed by immunological techniques [75]. A second test for activated clotting factors that must be performed according to the European Pharmacopoeia is the so-called non-activated partial thromboplastin time (NAPTT). Prescribed dilutions of PCC, phospholipids (blood platelet substitute), and calcium chloride are added to plasma anticoagulated with citrate and the time to clot formation is recorded. The test is valid when clotting time in the reference sample (with buffer instead of PCC) ranges between 200 and 350 s. PCC batches pass this test when clotting times are not less than 150 s. The NAPTT is extremely sensitive to activated factor IX (IXa). Release tests do not focus on activated factor VII (VIIa) and activated factor X (Xa). While 3F- and 4F-PCCs are virtually devoid of factor Xa, they do contain some factor VIIa [86]. Thrombotic complications, however, are a rare side effect of activated PCC (Feiba®) that contain substantial amounts of factor VIIa [87].

4. Mode of action

4.1. Vitamin K antagonists and reversal of anticoagulation by 4F-PCC

VKA anticoagulant coumarins like warfarin and phenprocoumon act by inhibiting the enzyme vitamin K reductase [88]. This enzymes shuffles vitamin K back into its active form. This "reactivated" vitamin K is needed to support the enzyme glutamylcarboxylase that converts glutamic acid residues into gamma glutamic acid (Gla) residues. During this process, vitamin K loses its activity again. Gla residues bind calcium-ions and this is essential for vitamin K-dependent coagulation factors to bind to negatively charged phospholipids and to partake in coagulation [89]. As a result of VKA therapy, fewer Gla residues are incorporated. The consequence of this is that circulating vitamin K-dependent coagulation factors are less functional. Upon triggering of the coagulation system, less prothrombin will be converted to

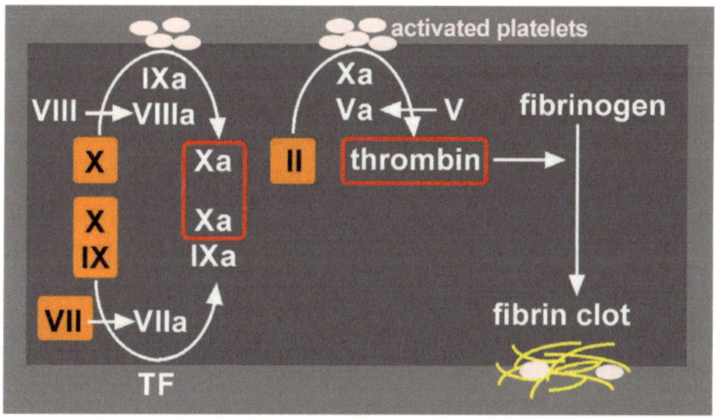

Figure 5. Anticoagulation targets and reversal of anticoagulation by 4F-PCC. Filled orange boxes indicate the vitamin K-dependent coagulation factors, targets for VKA therapy (vitamin K-dependent anticoagulant protein S and C are not depicted). Due to VKA therapy, vitamin K-dependent coagulation factors are synthesized with reduced procoagulant activity. Reversal of VKA anticoagulation by 4F-PCC infusion is accomplished by prompt replenishment of functional vitamin K-dependent coagulation factors. Red boxes indicate the NOAC targets. In NOAC-treated individuals, normal levels of fully functional clotting factors are to be expected. PCC infusion will increase the concentration of vitamin K-dependent coagulation factors above normal and more factor Xa and thrombin will be generated that escapes from NOAC inhibition, resulting in increased feedback amplification of the coagulation processes (see **Figure 1**). Similar mechanisms for VKA and NOAC reversal also apply to 3F-PCC (contains no factor VII) and activated PCC (contains factor VIIa instead of factor VII).

thrombin and time to clot formation will be markedly increased. Due to lower obtained levels of thrombin, also less thrombin-activatable fibrinolysis inhibitor (TAFI) will be activated. This inhibitor, once activated by thrombin, retards the clot lysis process. Thus, VKA therapy not only downscales clot formation but also enhances clot degradation [90].

Reversal of VKA anticoagulation can be done by cessation of VKA therapy together with the administration of vitamin K that boosts the synthesis of functional, Gla-domain-containing vitamin K-dependent coagulation factors [91, 92]. This "de novo" synthesis of coagulation factors, that takes place in the liver, may take too long. For immediate emergency reversal, replenishment of functional vitamin K-dependent clotting factors seems more appropriate. This can be achieved by intravenous administration of 4F-PCC (**Figure 5**).

4.2. Direct thrombin and factor Xa inhibitors and reversal of their anticoagulant action by 4F-PCC

Vitamin K-dependent coagulation factors circulate in plasma in their pro-enzymatic, inactive form. Enzymatic activity resides in their active center that is located in the catalytic domain (see **Figure 2**). In their pro-enzymatic form, the active center is shielded from interaction with target proteins. Direct thrombin and factor Xa inhibitor non-vitamin K oral anticoagulants (NOACs) are designed to target the respective active sites. Vitamin K administration is standard treatment to support VKA reversal by PCC. Obviously, in NOAC-treated individuals clotting factors are processed properly (normal posttranslational Gla residue incorporation) and hence vitamin K administration is usually not required. Cessation of NOAC therapy is one approach to reverse anticoagulation in NOAC-treated individuals. Due to the half-life of NOACs (5–17 h) [93], additional reversal measures may be needed in emergency situations.

4F-PCC can be used in situations requiring immediate reversal of anticoagulation by NOACs. Mechanism of action of PCC in NOAC reversal differs from that in VKA reversal (**Figure 5**). With respect to VKA reversal, PCC replenishes the level of functional vitamin K-dependent clotting factors. With regard to NOAC reversal, normal levels of fully functional clotting factors already are present in the circulation. The idea behind 4F-PCC as reversal agent for NOACs is that by increasing the concentration of vitamin K-dependent procoagulant factors, slightly more factor Xa and thrombin will be generated that escapes from inhibition by either a direct Xa or direct thrombin inhibitor resulting in increased feedback amplification of the coagulation processes [94]. This latter mechanism also underscores the general applicability of PCCs as an antidote for current and future direct oral anticoagulants.

5. Dosage, efficacy, and safety

5.1. PCC dosing for reversal of vitamin K antagonists

Despite decades of clinical experience with PCC, dosing is still a matter of debate [95]. The international normalized ratio or INR is a frequently used laboratory parameter to guide PCC dosing. This parameter is derived from the prothrombin time (PT) test. In this test, a plasma sample (citrate anticoagulated) is mixed with calcium-ions, tissue factor, and phospholipids and the time to clot formation is measured. The INR aims to harmonize PT results obtained with VKA-anticoagulated plasma regardless of the reagents and instrument used [4]. It should be noted, however, that PT to INR correction factors used for VKA-anticoagulated plasma do not apply for NOAC-anticoagulated plasma [96, 97]. INR values in normal individuals range between 0.8 and 1.2. The target level INR for people on VKA anticoagulation is usually between 2 and 3 [4]. In the "real world", INR values of 7 or higher can be observed as well. Target INR values for emergency reversal of anticoagulation vary between institutional protocols. A target INR of 1.3 or 1.5 is most often used [95].

PCC dosing strategies usually take into account the INR at presentation and the body weight of the patient. For example, 25 IU per kg body weight for a baseline INR < 4, 35 IU per kg for an INR between 4 and 6 and 50 IU per kg for an INR > 6. Other strategies also take into account the reason for which reversal by PCC is required [98, 99]. For example, a target INR of 2.1 for small urgent interventions and minor bleedings and a target INR of 1.5 for major bleeding [98]. More simplified regimens are also practiced, namely a fixed dose per individual (usually 1000 IU), a fixed dose per kg body weight (depending on the protocol ranging from 8 to 50 IU/kg), and a dose based on the clinical experience of the doctor. Relatively good INR outcomes were reported with the use of any treatment protocol while INR outcome in general was less satisfactory when a predefined protocol was missing (doctor strategy). Lowest PCC dosages will be infused in the fixed dose strategy [95].

Major advantage of a fixed dose per individual is a shorter time to infusion (median 130 min) as compared to strategies that require dosing calculation based on body weight and INR at presentation (median 160 min, p=0.015) [100]. One should also take into account that time is wasted between the first and, if clinically required, subsequent PCC infusions that may range between 1.5 and 8 hours [101]. In vitro spiking of plasma samples taken from VKA-treated individuals with increasing PCC dose has revealed INR normalization by 0.5 IU PCC per ml plasma, irrespective of the initial INR [101]. This value recalculates to a fixed dose of 20 IU/kg body weight or 1500 IU for a man with an average weight of 75 kg.

5.2. 4F-PCC versus plasma for rapid INR correction in VKA-anticoagulated individuals

Prospective studies in VKA-anticoagulated individuals have shown almost immediate INR correction after PCC infusion (6–83 IU/kg) and reached INR levels remained stable for at least 6 hours irrespective of the dosing regimen used [9, 11, 12, 98, 99, 102–105]. Infusion time of PCC is relatively low (7–75 min). This is in contrast to FFP, for which infusion times up to 900 min have been reported (**Table 3**) [11, 104, 105]. Importantly, infusion volume of PCC (25–320 ml) is considerably lower than that of FFP (350–1525 ml) [11, 12, 99, 102, 104]. Comparative prospective studies have revealed rapid INR reduction (INR ≤ 1.3 at 1 hour after start of the infusion) in 54–69% of individuals treated with PCC versus no patients in the plasma group [11, 12]. At the end of infusion, 55–100% of the patients treated with PCC had an INR of 1.3 or lower compared with no more than 10% of the patients treated with plasma instead (**Table 3**). Rapid INR reduction associated with the use of PCC, alone or as an adjunct to FFP, translates to a significant shorter time to invasive intervention in VKA patients requiring urgent surgery as compared to patients receiving FFP only [12, 106–109].

	PCC		FFP	
Reversal agent infusion				
- volume administered, ml	25-320	[11, 12, 99, 102, 104, 105]	353-1525	[11, 12]
- time to end of infusion, min	7-75	[11, 104, 105]	26-928	[11]
Clinical efficacy, % of study population				
- INR at target 1 hour after start infusion	54-69	[11, 12]	0	[11, 12]
- INR at target at end of infusion	55-100	[9, 11, 12, 99, 102–105]	0-10	[9, 11, 12]
- hemostatic efficacy, good or excellent	72-100	[11, 12, 99, 103, 105]	65-75	[11, 12]
Adverse events, % of study population(treatment related)				
- volume overload	0-5	[11, 12, 13]	7-13	[11-13]
- thromboembolic complications	2-8 (2-3)	[102, 104, 105, 110]	8 (3)	[110]
- mortality	1-19 (0-2)	[99, 102–105, 110]	13 (2)	[110]

Table 3. Comparison of FFP with 4F-PCC for the reversal of warfarin anticoagulation.

5.3. INR versus clinical efficacy

The INR is the outcome of standardized laboratory testing and is a tool to monitor VKA treatment and to guide reversal by PCC. Effective hemostasis or clinical efficacy is usually defined as a rating of excellent or good as judged by the attending physician and is confirmed when no additional measures are needed to maintain normal hemostasis in patients needing urgent surgical or invasive interventions, or when visual bleeding has stopped, no further decrease in hemoglobin is observed, blood pressure is normalized, and no further PCC or blood transfusion (plasma or red blood cells) is required in patients presenting with major bleeding. INR at end point and clinical efficacy, thus, are different albeit related parameters. It should be noted that the choice of a target INR is arbitrary, with no clear clinical proof for the advantage of a low target INR. Obviously, choosing a high INR target will result in a higher relative number of individuals reaching this target. For example, a study among 103 PCC-treated VKA patients revealed that 86 patients (83.5%) had an excellent clinical response (control of bleeding, no additional hemostatic measures required) while only 50 patients (48.5%) had a final INR response of ≤ 1.5. On the other hand, 95 patients (92.2%) were on target when an INR of 2.0 was considered [111]. Thus, clinical efficacy may serve as a more reliable measure for the usefulness of PCC in VKA reversal than the percentage of individuals reaching a certain INR target. It is worth mentioning that the INR is neither a reliable predictor of hemorrhage nor an appropriate guide for PCC dosing strategies [101, 112–114]. Nevertheless, the INR remains a useful tool to monitor VKA treatment and reversal of anticoagulation [114].

5.4. Clinical efficacy of 4F-PCC for rapid VKA reversal: influence of dosing regimen

The question seems relevant whether different dosing regimens result in different clinical outcomes. Using initial INR and body weight-guided dosing regimen (25, 35, and 50 IU/kg for baseline INR of 2–3, 4–6, or > 6 respectively), good to excellent hemostasis was observed in 72–100% of the included individuals [11, 12, 102, 104, 105]. Studies with dosing regimens also including the target INR show similar clinical outcome [98, 100]. An observational, prospective, two-cohort Dutch comparison of a fixed 1000 IU versus variable dosing strategy (dosing based on patient body weight, baseline INR and target INR) revealed a successful clinical outcome in 96 and 88% of the included patients, respectively. This study thus shows a slight albeit significant (p=0.015) beneficial effect of a fixed dose of 1000 IU over variable dosing [100]. In a recent retrospective Canadian study, a total of 103 patients requiring urgent warfarin reversal were treated with PCC at a single fixed dose of 1000 IU. Excellent clinical response was observed in 83% of treated patients [111]. Based on higher expected patient weight, a US trauma center used a fixed dose of 1500 IU with a successful clinical outcome of 80% [115]. A systematic review including 27 studies revealed no clear evidence that one dosing strategy is superior [95]. Studies so far performed on clinical outcome have disregarded compositional differences between PCC products (see **Table 2**). Whether heparin-free PCC is of clinical benefit thus remains to be established. Differences between clinical outcome and cause of required VKA reversal, either a major bleeding or the need for urgent surgical intervention, are not reported. Given the shorter time to PCC infusion when using a fixed dose regimen compared to variable dosing, fixed dosing of 1000–1500 IU 4F-PCC may be preferred. Concurrent laboratory testing on patient's baseline plasma sample could then be used to guide additional PCC treatment.

5.5. 4F-PCC dosing for effective reversal of direct thrombin and factor Xa inhibitors

Clinical experience regarding the effectiveness and implementation of 4F-PCC in the treatment of NOAC-associated bleeds is limited. Though there have been several studies of NOAC reversal in healthy volunteers that focus on normalization of certain in vitro laboratory parameters [38, 116–119], well-designed randomized controlled clinical trials aiming at bleeding cessation measurements are difficult to perform in this setting. Most studies on the hemostatic effectiveness of PCC in NOAC reversal therefore have been performed in animal bleeding models (**Table 4**). One elegant double-blind, randomized, placebo-controlled study has explored the reversal of edoxaban by 4F-PCC in human volunteers using the punch biopsy bleeding model [38]. A total of 110 subjects were treated. Intravenous administration of 4F-PCC at a dose of 50, 25, or 10 IU/kg following administration of edoxaban (60 mg) dose-dependently reversed edoxaban's effects on bleeding duration, with complete reversal at 50 IU/kg. A similar dose-dependent reversal of edoxaban-associated bleeding by 4F-PCC was observed in rabbits following kidney incision [39]. The same bleeding model was used to demonstrate successful reversal of apixaban- as well as rivaroxaban-associated bleeds [37, 40]. In the aforementioned study, reversal by PCC was examined at different rivaroxaban concentrations. Low dose rivaroxaban (0.15 mg/kg) was almost completely reversed by low dose 4F-PCC (25 IU/kg). Intermediate rivaroxaban dose (0.30 mg/kg) required four times as much PCC (100 IU/kg) to obtain a similar reversal effect, while high dose rivaroxaban (0.45 mg/kg) could not be reversed [40]. This observation clearly illustrates a NOAC concentration dependent reversal by PCC. Two studies showed unsuccessful reversal of apixaban and rivaroxaban anticoagulation, that may relate to the bleeding model used (poly trauma) as well as to the NOAC and PCC dose administered [43, 44]. Dabigatran has been examined in six different animal bleeding models (**Table 4**). One study using PCC at a dose of 14 IU/kg did not reveal any improvement in dabigatran-associated hemorrhage [32]. The 5 other studies however showed partial to complete correction of dabigatran-associated bleeds [41, 42, 46, 48, 49]. The general consensus emerging from these studies is that a PCC dose ≤ 25 IU/kg is too low to be successful. Almost complete to complete correction of NOAC-associated bleeds requires a PCC dose of at least 50 IU/kg.

Study	Bleeding model	NOAC	PCC, IU/kg		Correction of blood loss (BL)/ bleeding time (BT)
[43]	Rabbit, poly trauma	Apixaban 0.4 mg/kg single bolus iv + 0.6 mg/kg.h continuous infusion iv	Kanokad	100	no / partial
[37]	Rabbit, kidney incision	Apixaban 1.2 mg/kg single dose iv	Beriplex	100 25 6	almost complete almost complete partial
[38]	Human, skin biopsy	Edoxaban 60 mg single dose orally	Beriplex	50 25 10	complete partial no
[39]	Rabbit, kidney incision	Edoxaban 1.2 mg/kg single dose iv	Beriplex	75 50 25	almost complete partial no
[44]	Rabbit, poly trauma	Rivaroxaban 5 mg/kg single dose iv	Kaskadil	40	no
[45]	Rat, small artery incision	Rivaroxaban 2 mg/kg single dose iv	Beriplex	50 25	almost complete (no BL data) no (no BL data)
[40]	Rabbit, kidney incision	Rivaroxaban single dose iv 0.45 mg/kg 0.30 mg/kg 0.30 mg/kg 0.30 mg/kg 0.15 mg/kg	Beriplex	100 100 50 25 25	no almost complete partial no almost complete
[47]	Mouse, intracerebral hemorrhage	Rivaroxaban 30 mg/kg single dose orally	Beriplex	100	almost complete (no BT data)
[46]	Mouse, tail bleeding and intracerebral hemorrhage	Dabigatran etexilate 9 mg/kg single dose ip	Beriplex	100 50 25	almost complete partial partial
[32]	Mouse, tail bleeding	Dabigatran etexilate 60 mg/kg single dose orally	Octaplex	14	no
[41]	Rabbit, kidney incision	Dabigatran 0.4 mg/kg single dose iv	Beriplex	50 20	complete/almost complete partial
[48]	Rat, tail bleeding	Dabigatran etexilate 30 mg/kg single dose orally	Beriplex	50 20	almost complete (no BL data) partial (no BL data)
[42]	Pig, poly trauma	Dabigatran etexilate 30 mg/kg bid (3d) orally + dabigatran 0.5 mg/kg iv prior trauma	Beriplex	100 50 25	yes* (no BT data) yes* (no BT data) no (no BT data)
[49]	Mouse, saphenous vein incision	Dabigatran 0.015 mg/kg single iv dose	Beriplex	50 25	complete (no BL data) no (no BL data)

*Data on bleeding tendency in normal, not NOAC treated animals was not provided in the study report. iv, intravenous. ip, intraperitoneal.

Table 4. NOAC reversal by 4F-PCC *in vivo*: effect on bleeding diathesis.

http://dx.doi.org/10.5772/64304

5.6. Safety profile of PCC

PCCs may have a better safety profile than FFP. Freeze-dried 4F-PCC products can be reconstituted in a small volume of diluent. Due to the small volume of the reconstituted product, PCCs can be administered in shorter infusion times with lower risk of volume overload than FFP [13]. Importantly, there is minimal risk of transfusion-related acute lung injury as PCCs lack anti-human leukocyte antigen/anti-granulocyte antibodies [120]. PCCs carry a negligible risk for viral transmission due to the incorporation of viral reduction steps in the manufacturing process. PCCs in contrast to FFP do not need AB0 typing. Adverse events associated with the use of PCC may include heparin-induced thrombocytopenia type II for those brands that contain heparin [121]. One retrospective study reported a slight increased risk of acute kidney injury associated with PCC as compared to FFP [122]. Mortality and thrombogenic events such as stroke, myocardial infarction, pulmonary embolism, disseminated intravascular coagulation, and deep vein thrombosis in cohorts treated with either FFP or PCC are similar (**Table 3**).

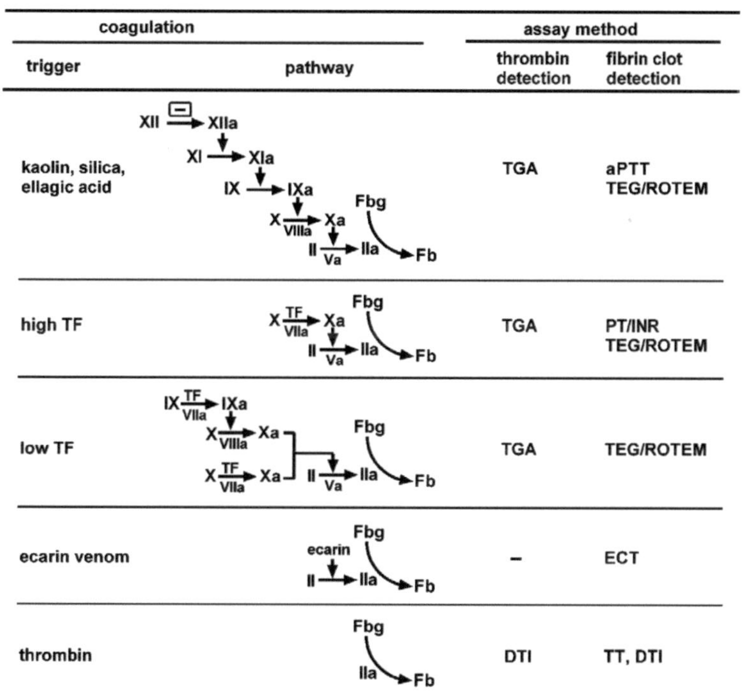

Figure 6. Coagulation assay methods. Global coagulation assays are either based on the measurement of thrombin or on the measurement of fibrin. aPTT is triggered by a negatively charged surface like kaolin, as such facilitating the contact activation pathway (intrinsic coagulation). Kaolin, silica, or ellagic acid triggering can also be used in TGA and TEG/ROTEM. Tissue factor (TF) triggering facilitates the extrinsic coagulation pathway. PT/INR is triggered by high TF concentrations, a condition that also can be used in TGA and TEG/ROTEM. Low TF concentration improves sensitivity, a condition frequently applied in TGA and TEG/ROTEM. The ecarin clotting time (ECT) is triggered by the venom from viper *Echis carinatus*. The thrombin time (TT) and direct thrombin inhibitor test (DTI) are both triggered by thrombin.

6. Reversal assessment by laboratory coagulation assays

6.1. Global coagulation tests

Global coagulation assays are most suited for the assessment of reversal of anticoagulation [114]. Global coagulation tests do not pinpoint any specific coagulation factor but instead generate data on the coagulation potential of a plasma sample as a whole. Global coagulation tests focus either on the generation of thrombin (thrombin generation assay, TGA) or on the generation of fibrin clots (PT, aPTT, ROTEM, TEG). PT and aPTT are clotting time based assays, while ROTEM (rotational thromboelastometry) and TEG (thromboelastograpy) also generate data on kinetics of clot formation, clot strength, and clot stability. Sensitivity of global assays for certain coagulation factors is determined by the choice and concentration of the coagulation trigger used (see **Figure 6** and reference [114]).

6.2. Monitoring PCC treatment in VKA-anticoagulated individuals

The contact activation-triggered aPTT in general is less sensitive to VKA treatment than the TF-triggered PT test [114]. This is probably due to the fact that the aPTT does not detect variations in factor VII, the most significant vitamin K-dependent clotting factor in determining the PT outcome in VKA-anticoagulated plasma [123]. The PT with its derived international normalized ratio (INR) is worldwide the most commonly used assay to monitor VKA treatment and reversal of anticoagulation by PCC. TF-triggered TEG/ROTEM and TGA also show good sensitivity to assess VKA anticoagulation and reversal thereof [101, 114].

6.3. Monitoring PCC treatment in NOAC-anticoagulated individuals

NOACs may affect any assay that depends on factor Xa or IIa (thrombin) activity, including the PT, aPTT, TGA, and TEG/TEM (see **Figure 6** and reference [114]). Two other clotting time based tests, the thrombin time (TT) and ecarin clotting time (ECT) are affected in particular by direct thrombin inhibitors. Sensitivity of a certain test to NOACs, however, does not directly mean that the test is suitable to assess reversal of anticoagulation by PCC. For example, clotting in the TT test is triggered by adding excess thrombin to a plasma sample, as such overruling the complete coagulation cascade (see **Figure 6**). As a consequence, dabigatran in the plasma sample will inhibit the added thrombin without being affected by increased clotting factor levels due to PCC administration. Likewise, PCC administration will be unnoticed in the ECT test in which coagulation in a sample is triggered by snake venom that completely converts prothrombin into thrombin [114]. Similarly, assays that are triggered by the addition of excess factor Xa (e.g. anti-Xa assays designed for rivaroxaban determinations) will not reveal reversal of anticoagulation by clotting factor concentrates.

The most promising assay parameter to reveal reversal of NOAC anticoagulation by PCC infusion is the area under the thrombin generation curve (TGA-AUC or ETP). The PT is less sensitive while the aPTT is insensitive in this respect [94, 114, 124]. Zahir et al. have explored the reversal of edoxaban by 4F-PCC in human volunteers using the punch biopsy bleeding model [38]. The effect of 4F-PCC on TGA-ETP was similar to the effects on bleeding duration

http://dx.doi.org/10.5772/64304

and bleeding volume, suggesting that TGA-ETP is an appropriate surrogate biomarker for assessing the effect on bleeding. Several studies on NOAC reversal by PCC in healthy human volunteers have used the TGA-AUC as outcome measure, showing partial to complete normalization 30 min post dose (**Table 5**). Of note is the observed overcorrection of TGA-AUC 24 hours post dose that can be explained by a relative short half-life of NOACs as compared to PCC.

Study	NOAC	PCC, IU/kg		Correction of TGA-AUC	
				30 min Post dose	24 hour Post dose
[118]	Apixaban	Cofact	37	Partial	Overcorrection
	10 mg bid, 2.5 days		25	Partial	Overcorrection
[38]	Edoxaban	Beriplex	50	Complete	Overcorrection
	60 mg single dose		25	Partial	Overcorrection
			10	No	No
[116]	Rivaroxaban	Cofact	50	Complete	Overcorrection
	20 mg bid, 2.5 days				
[119]	Rivaroxaban	Cofact	37	Partial	Overcorrection
	15 mg bid, 2.5 days		25	Partial	Complete
[117]	Rivaroxaban	Beriplex	50	Partial	Overcorrection
	20 mg bid, 5.5 days	Profilnine	50	Partial	Overcorrection

Effect on ex vivo thrombin generation in healthy human volunteers.

Table 5. NOAC reversal by PCC *in vivo*.

7. Concluding remarks

Clinical emergency situations may require rapid reversal of anticoagulation. 4F-PCC seems very suitable to reverse VKA as well as NOAC anticoagulation. Activated PCC can also be used. 3F-PCC seems less effective in the reversal of VKA anticoagulation. Several laboratory assays are suited for monitoring VKA reversal, including the INR as well as other global assays such as thrombin generation and thromboelastography. As to NOAC reversal monitoring, one should be aware of the fact that several laboratory assays including direct thrombin and direct factor Xa inhibitor assay do not reveal an increase in procoagulant potential upon PCC infusion. The ETP seems an appropriate biomarker for assessing the effect of PCC administration on NOAC anticoagulation. In contrast, PT is less sensitive and the aPTT is insensitive in this respect.

Clinically effective reversal of VKA anticoagulation can be obtained with the use of any treatment protocol. Time till PCC infusion and consequently time till follow up treatment can be shorted by prompt infusion of a fixed dose of 1000–1500 IU 4F-PCC per individual, irrespective of INR at presentation, target INR, and body weight. For NOAC reversal, at least 50 IU/kg or 4000 IU for a body weight of 80 kg seems required. Its non-specific nature is a major advantage of PCC over specific agents that block NOACs. PCCs can readily be infused, while specific NOAC antidotes require the need for laborious anticoagulant identification prior to antidote selection and administration. PCCs also are probably cheaper and more widely available in general hospitals than specific NOAC antidotes. Some PCCs are supplemented with heparin that may counteract the prohemostatic effect of the PCC. Safety profile of PCC is similar to that of FFP.

8. Conflict of interest statement

The author is employee of Sanquin Research, a division of Sanquin. Sanquin is manufacturer of 4-factor PCC (Cofact®).

Author details

Herm Jan M. Brinkman

Address all correspondence to: h.brinkman@sanquin.nl

Department of Plasma Proteins, Sanquin Research, Amsterdam, The Netherlands

References

[1] Furie B, Furie BC. Mechanisms of thrombus formation. N Engl J Med. 2008;359:938–949.

[2] Mackman N. The role of tissue factor and factor VIIa in hemostasis. Anesth Analg. 2009;108:1447–1452.

[3] Mann KG. Thrombin generation in hemorrhage control and vascular occlusion. Circulation. 2011;124:225–235.

[4] Ageno W, Gallus AS, Wittkowsky A, Crowther M, Hylek EM, Palareti G; American College of Chest Physicians. Oral anticoagulant therapy: antithrombotic therapy and prevention of thrombosis, 9th ed: American College of Chest Physicians Evidence-Based Clinical Practice Guidelines. Chest. 2012;141(2 Suppl):e44S–88S.

[5] Anand SS, Yusuf S. Oral anticoagulant therapy in patients with coronary artery disease: a meta-analysis. JAMA. 1999;282:2058–2067.

[6] Eerenberg ES, Middeldorp S, Levi M, Lensing AW, Büller HR. Clinical impact and course of major bleeding with rivaroxaban and vitamin K antagonists. J Thromb Haemost. 2015;13:1590–1596.

[7] Graham DJ, Reichman ME, Wernecke M, Zhang R, Southworth MR, Levenson M, Sheu TC, Mott K, Goulding MR, Houstoun M, MaCurdy TE, Worrall C, Kelman JA. Cardiovascular, bleeding, and mortality risks in elderly Medicare patients treated with dabigatran or warfarin for nonvalvular atrial fibrillation. Circulation. 2015;131:157–164.

[8] Fredriksson K, Norrving B, Strömblad LG. Emergency reversal of anticoagulation after intracerebral hemorrhage. Stroke. 1992;23:972–977.

[9] Makris M, Greaves M, Phillips WS, Kitchen S, Rosendaal FR, Preston EF. Emergency oral anticoagulant reversal: the relative efficacy of infusions of fresh frozen plasma and clotting factor concentrate on correction of the coagulopathy. Thromb Haemost. 1997;77:477–480.

[10] Wójcik C, Schymik ML, Cure EG. Activated prothrombin complex concentrate factor VIII inhibitor bypassing activity (FEIBA) for the reversal of warfarin-induced coagulopathy. Int J Emerg Med. 2009;2:217–225.

[11] Sarode R, Milling TJ Jr, Refaai MA, Mangione A, Schneider A, Durn BL, Goldstein JN. Efficacy and safety of a 4-factor prothrombin complex concentrate in patients on vitamin K antagonists presenting with major bleeding: a randomized, plasma-controlled, phase IIIb study. Circulation. 2013;128:1234–1243.

[12] Goldstein JN, Refaai MA, Milling TJ Jr, Lewis B, Goldberg-Alberts R, Hug BA, Sarode R. Four-factor prothrombin complex concentrate versus plasma for rapid vitamin K antagonist reversal in patients needing urgent surgical or invasive interventions: a phase 3b, open-label, non-inferiority, randomised trial. Lancet. 2015;385:2077–2087.

[13] Refaai MA, Goldstein JN, Lee ML, Durn BL, Milling TJ Jr, Sarode R. Increased risk of volume overload with plasma compared with four-factor prothrombin complex concentrate for urgent vitamin K antagonist reversal. Transfusion. 2015;55:2722–2729.

[14] Menache D. Coagulation factor concentrate: historical perspective. Haemophilia. 1995;1:7–12.

[15] Hanley JP. Warfarin reversal. J Clin Pathol. 2004;57:1132–1139.

[16] Leissinger CA, Blatt PM, Hoots WK, Ewenstein B. Role of prothrombin complex concentrates in reversing warfarin anticoagulation: a review of the literature. Am J Hematol. 2008;83:137–143.

[17] Unold D, Tormey CA. Clinical applications of 4-factor prothrombin complex concentrate: a practical pathologist's perspective. Arch Pathol Lab Med. 2015;139:1568–1575.

[18] Holland L, Warkentin TE, Refaai M, Crowther MA, Johnston MA, Sarode R. Suboptimal effect of a three-factor prothrombin complex concentrate (Profilnine-SD) in correcting supratherapeutic international normalized ratio due to warfarin overdose. Transfusion. 2009;49:1171–1177.

[19] Voils SA, Baird B. Systematic review: 3-factor versus 4-factor prothrombin complex concentrate for warfarin reversal: does it matter? Thromb Res. 2012;130:833–840.

[20] Voils SA, Holder MC, Premraj S, Catlin JR, Allen BR. Comparative effectiveness of 3- versus 4-factor prothrombin complex concentrate for emergent warfarin reversal. Thromb Res. 2015;136:595–598.

[21] Al-Majzoub O, Rybak E, Reardon DP, Krause P, Connors JM. Evaluation of warfarin reversal with 4-factor prothrombin complex concentrate compared to 3-factor prothrombin complex concentrate at a tertiary academic medical center. J Emerg Med. 2016;50:7–13.

[22] Stewart WS, Pettit H. Experiences with an activated 4-factor prothrombin complex concentrate (FEIBA) for reversal of warfarin-related bleeding. Am J Emerg Med. 2013;31:1251–1254.

[23] Yank V, Tuohy CV, Logan AC, Bravata DM, Staudenmayer K, Eisenhut R, Sundaram V, McMahon D, Olkin I, McDonald KM, Owens DK, Stafford RS. Systematic review: benefits and harms of in-hospital use of recombinant factor VIIa for off-label indications. Ann Intern Med. 2011;154:529–540.

[24] Brody DL, Aiyagari V, Shackleford AM, Diringer MN. Use of recombinant factor VIIa in patients with warfarin-associated intracranial hemorrhage. Neurocrit Care. 2005;2:263–267.

[25] Nishijima DK, Dager WE, Schrot RJ, Holmes JF. The efficacy of factor VIIa in emergency department patients with warfarin use and traumatic intracranial hemorrhage. Acad Emerg Med. 2010;17:244–251.

[26] Chou SHY, Xuemei C, Konigsberg RG, Bresette LM, van Galen H, Fazaneh SA, Steven KF. Thromboembolic risks of recombinant factor VIIa use in warfarin-associated intracranial hemorrhage: a case-control study. BMC Neurol. 2012;12:158.

[27] DeLoughery EP, Lenfesty B, DeLoughery TG. The use of recombinant factor VIIa in warfarin patients with traumatic brain injury: a retrospective case-control study. Blood Coagul Fibrinolysis. 2013;24:317–320.

[28] Sarode R, Matevosyan K, Bhagat R, Rutherford C, Madden C, Beshay JE. Rapid warfarin reversal: a 3-factor prothrombin complex concentrate and recombinant factor VIIa cocktail for intracerebral hemorrhage. J Neurosurg. 2012;116:491–497.

[29] Weeterings C, de Groot PG, Adelmeijer J, Lisman T. The glycoprotein Ib-IX-V complex contributes to tissue factor-independent thrombin generation by recombinant factor VIIa on the activated platelet surface. Blood. 2008;112:3227–3233.

[30] Dickneite G. Prothrombin complex concentrate versus recombinant factor VIIa for reversal of coumarin anticoagulation. Thromb Res. 2007;119:643–651.

[31] Skolnick BE, Mathews DR, Khutoryansky NM, Pusateri AE, Carr ME. Exploratory study on the reversal of warfarin with rFVIIa in healthy subjects. Blood. 2010;116:693–701.

[32] Lambourne MD, Eltringham-Smith LJ, Gataiance S, Arnold DM, Crowther MA, Sheffield WP. Prothrombin complex concentrates reduce blood loss in murine coagulopathy induced by warfarin, but not in that induced by dabigatran etexilate. J Thromb Haemost. 2012;10:1830–1840.

[33] Schlunk F, Van Cott EM, Hayakawa K, Pfeilschifter W, Lo EH, Foerch C. Recombinant activated coagulation factor VII and prothrombin complex concentrates are equally effective in reducing hematoma volume in experimental warfarin-associated intracerebral hemorrhage. Stroke. 2012;43:246–249.

[34] Illanes S, Zhou W, Schwarting S, Heiland S, Veltkamp R. Comparative effectiveness of hemostatic therapy in experimental warfarin-associated intracerebral hemorrhage. Stroke. 2011;42:191–195.

[35] Franchini M, Bonfanti C, Mannucci PM. Management of bleeding associated with new oral anticoagulants. Semin Thromb Hemost. 2015;41:788–801.

[36] Crowther M, Crowther MA. Antidotes for novel oral anticoagulants: current status and future potential. Arterioscler Thromb Vasc Biol. 2015;35:1736–1745.

[37] Herzog E, Kaspereit F, Krege W, Mueller-Cohrs J, Doerr B, Niebl P, Dickneite G. Four-factor prothrombin complex concentrate reverses apixaban-associated bleeding in a rabbit model of acute hemorrhage. J Thromb Haemost. 2015;13:2220–2226.

[38] Zahir H, Brown KS, Vandell AG, Desai M, Maa JF, Dishy V, Lomeli B, Feussner A, Feng W, He L, Grosso MA, Lanz HJ, Antman EM. Edoxaban effects on bleeding following punch biopsy and reversal by a 4-factor prothrombin complex concentrate. Circulation. 2015;131:82–90.

[39] Herzog E, Kaspereit F, Krege W, Doerr B, Mueller-Cohrs J, Pragst I, Morishima Y, Dickneite G. Effective reversal of edoxaban-associated bleeding with four-factor prothrombin complex concentrate in a rabbit model of acute hemorrhage. Anesthesiology. 2015;122:387–398.

[40] Herzog E, Kaspereit F, Krege W, Mueller-Cohrs J, Doerr B, Niebl P, Dickneite G. Correlation of coagulation markers and 4F-PCC-mediated reversal of rivaroxaban in a rabbit model of acute bleeding. Thromb Res. 2015;135:554–560.

[41] Pragst I, Zeitler SH, Doerr B, Kaspereit FJ, Herzog E, Dickneite G, van Ryn J. Reversal of dabigatran anticoagulation by prothrombin complex concentrate (Beriplex P/N) in a rabbit model. J Thromb Haemost. 2012;10:1841–1848.

[42] Honickel M, Braunschweig T, van Ryn J, Ten Cate H, Spronk HM, Rossaint R, Grottke O. Prothrombin complex concentrate is effective in treating the anticoagulant effects of dabigatran in a porcine polytrauma model. Anesthesiology. 2015;123:1350–1361.

[43] Martin AC, Le Bonniec B, Fischer AM, Marchand-Leroux C, Gaussem P, Samama CM, Godier A. Evaluation of recombinant activated factor VII, prothrombin complex concentrate, and fibrinogen concentrate to reverse apixaban in a rabbit model of bleeding and thrombosis. Int J Cardiol. 2013;168:4228–4233.

[44] Godier A, Miclot A, Le Bonniec B, Durand M, Fischer AM, Emmerich J, Marchand-Leroux C, Lecompte T, Samama CM. Evaluation of prothrombin complex concentrate and recombinant activated factor VII to reverse rivaroxaban in a rabbit model. Anesthesiology. 2012;116:94–102.

[45] Perzborn E, Gruber A, Tinel H, Marzec UM, Buetehorn U, Buchmueller A, Heitmeier S, Laux V. Reversal of rivaroxaban anticoagulation by haemostatic agents in rats and primates. Thromb Haemost. 2013;110:162–172.

[46] Zhou W, Schwarting S, Illanes S, Liesz A, Middelhoff M, Zorn M, Bendszus M, Heiland S, van Ryn J, Veltkamp R. Hemostatic therapy in experimental intracerebral hemorrhage associated with the direct thrombin inhibitor dabigatran. Stroke. 2011;42:3594–3599.

[47] Zhou W, Zorn M, Nawroth P, Bütehorn U, Perzborn E, Heitmeier S, Veltkamp R. Hemostatic therapy in experimental intracerebral hemorrhage associated with rivaroxaban. Stroke. 2013;44:771–778.

[48] van Ryn J, Schurer J, Kink-Eiband M, Clemens A. Reversal of dabigatran-induced bleeding by coagulation factor concentrates in a rat-tail bleeding model and lack of effect on assays of coagulation. Anesthesiology. 2014;120:1429–1440.

[49] Hoffman M, Volovyk Z, Monroe DM. Reversal of dabigatran effects in models of thrombin generation and hemostasis by factor VIIa and prothrombin complex concentrate. Anesthesiology. 2015;122:353–362.

[50] Honickel M, Maron B, van Ryn J, Braunschweig T, Ten Cate H, Spronk HM, Rossaint R, Grottke O. Therapy with activated prothrombin complex concentrate is effective in reducing dabigatran-associated blood loss in a porcine polytrauma model. Thromb Haemost. 2016;115:271–284.

[51] Ross B, Miller MA, Ditch K, Tran M. Clinical experience of life-threatening dabigatran-related bleeding at a large, tertiary care, academic medical center: a case series. J Med Toxicol. 2014;10:223–228.

[52] Beyer-Westendorf J, Förster K, Pannach S, Ebertz F, Gelbricht V, Thieme C, Michalski F, Köhler C, Werth S, Sahin K, Tittl L, Hänsel U, Weiss N. Rates, management, and outcome of rivaroxaban bleeding in daily care: results from the Dresden NOAC registry. Blood. 2014;124:955–962.

[53] Grandhi R, Newman WC, Zhang X, Harrison G, Moran C, Okonkwo DO, Ducruet AF. Administration of 4-factor prothrombin complex concentrate as an antidote for intracranial bleeding in patients taking direct factor Xa inhibitors. World Neurosurg. 2015;84:1956–1961.

[54] Dibu JR, Weimer JM, Ahrens C, Manno E, Frontera JA. The role of FEIBA in reversing novel oral anticoagulants in intracerebral hemorrhage. Neurocrit Care. 2016;24:413-419. Doi: 10.1007/s12028-015-0213-y.

[55] Hagen FS, Gray CL, O'Hara P, Grant FJ, Saari GC, Woodbury RG, Hart CE, Insley M, Kisiel W, Kurachi K, et al. Characterization of a cDNA coding for human factor VII. Proc Natl Acad Sci USA. 1986;83:2412–2416.

[56] Chen SW, Pellequer JL, Schved JF, Giansily-Blaizot M. Model of a ternary complex between activated factor VII, tissue factor and factor IX. Thromb Haemost. 2002;88:74–82.

[57] Leytus SP, Foster DC, Kurachi K, Davie EW. Gene for human factor X: a blood coagulation factor whose gene organization is essentially identical with that of factor IX and protein C. Biochemistry. 1986;25:5098–5102.

[58] Yoshitake S, Schach BG, Foster DC, Davie EW, Kurachi K. Nucleotide sequence of the gene for human factor IX (antihemophilic factor B). Biochemistry. 1985;24:3736–3750.

[59] Shikamoto Y, Morita T, Fujimoto Z, Mizuno H. Crystal structure of Mg2+- and Ca2+-bound Gla domain of factor IX complexed with binding protein. J Biol Chem. 2003;278:24090–24094.

[60] Degen SJ, Davie EW. Nucleotide sequence of the gene for human prothrombin. Biochemistry. 1987;26:6165–6177.

[61] Pozzi N, Chen Z, Gohara DW, Niu W, Heyduk T, Di Cera E. Crystal structure of prothrombin reveals conformational flexibility and mechanism of activation. J Biol Chem. 2013;288:22734–22744.

[62] Davie EW, Kulman JD. An overview of the structure and function of thrombin. Semin Thromb Hemost. 2006;32 Suppl 1:3–15.

[63] Foster DC, Yoshitake S, Davie EW. The nucleotide sequence of the gene for human protein C. Proc Natl Acad Sci USA. 1985;82:4673–4677.

[64] Dahlbäck B, Villoutreix BO. Regulation of blood coagulation by the protein C anticoagulant pathway: novel insights into structure-function relationships and molecular recognition. Arterioscler Thromb Vasc Biol. 2005;25:1311–1320.

[65] Lundwall A, Dackowski W, Cohen E, Shaffer M, Mahr A, Dahlbäck B, Stenflo J, Wydro R. Isolation and sequence of the cDNA for human protein S, a regulator of blood coagulation. Proc Natl Acad Sci USA. 1986;83:6716–6720.

[66] Köhler M. Thrombogenicity of prothrombin complex concentrates. Thromb Res. 1999;95(Suppl 1):S13–7.

[67] Grundman C, Plesker R, Kusch M, Hanschmann KM, Eich S, Seitz R, König H. Prothrombin overload causes thromboembolic complications in prothrombin complex concentrates: in vitro and in vivo evidence. Thromb Haemost. 2005;94:1338–1339.

[68] Hellstern P. Production and composition of prothrombin complex concentrates: correlation between composition and therapeutic efficiency. Thromb Res 1999;95(4 Suppl 1):S7–12.

[69] Josic D, Hoffer L, Buchacher A. Preparation of vitamin K-dependent proteins, such as clotting factors II, VII, IX and X and clotting inhibitor protein C. J Chromatogr B Analyt Technol Biomed Life Sci. 2003;790:183–197.

[70] Brigulla M, Thiele T, Scharf C, Breitner-Ruddock S, Venz S, Völker U, Greinacher A. Proteomics as a tool for assessment of therapeutics in transfusion medicine: evaluation of prothrombin complex concentrates. Transfusion. 2006;46:377–385.

[71] Okutucu B, Dinçer A, Habib O, Zihnioglu F. Comparison of five methods for determination of total plasma protein concentration. J Biochem Biophys Methods. 2007;70:709–711.

[72] Blombäck M, Abildgaard U, van den Besselaar AM, Clementson KJ, Dahlbäck B, Exner T, Francis CW, Gaffney P, Gralnick H, Hoyer LW, et al. Nomenclature of quantities and units in thrombosis and haemostasis (recommendation 1993). A collaborative project of the scientific and standardization committee of the International Society on Thrombosis and Haemostasis (ISTH/SSC) and the Commission/Committee on Quantities and Units (in Clinical Chemistry) of the International Union of Pure and Applied Chemistry-International Federation of Clinical Chemistry (IUPAC-IFCC/CQU(CC)). Thromb Haemost 1994;71:375–394.

[73] Brinkman HJ, Patiwael S, Tripathi S, Meijers JC. Heparin supplement counteracts the prohemostatic effect of prothrombin complex concentrate and factor IX concentrate: an in vitro evaluation. Thromb Res. 2016;139:102–110.

[74] Kalina U, Bickhard H, Schulte S. Biochemical comparison of seven commercially available prothrombin complex concentrates. Int J Clin Pract. 2008;62:1614–1622.

[75] Sadeghi N, Kahn D, Sayed D, Hoppenstadt D, Jeske W, Harenberg J, Dechristopher P, Fareed J. Compositional differences in commercially available prothrombin complex concentrates. Clin Appl Thromb Hemost. 2014;20:256–269.

[76] Grottke O, Rossaint R, Henskens Y, van Oerle R, Ten Cate H, Spronk HM. Thrombin generation capacity of prothrombin complex concentrate in an in vitro dilutional model. PLoS One 2013;8:e64100.

[77] Sørensen B, Spahn DR, Innerhofer P, Spannagl M, Rossaint R. Clinical review: prothrombin complex concentrates – evaluation of safety and thrombogenicity. Crit Care. 2011;15:201.

[78] Hemker HC, Al Dieri R, De Smedt E, Béguin S. Thrombin generation, a function test of the haemostatic-thrombotic system. Thromb Haemost. 2006;96:553–561.

[79] Takeyama M, Sakurai Y, Shima M, Matsumoto T, Nogami K, Tanaka I, Takeda T, Giddings JC, Yoshioka A. Heparin-induced inhibitory effects of a prothrombin complex concentrate on global tests of haemostasis. Blood Coagul Fibrinolysis. 2007;18:1–7.

[80] Scharbert G, Thaler U, Weilnböck C, Wetzel L, Kozek-Langenecker S. Heparin-induced effects of prothrombin complex concentrates in thromboelastometry. Wien Klin Wochenschr. 2012;124:320–325.

[81] Felli A, Zeidler P, Jilma B, Opfermann P, Caroline Holaubek, Zimpfer D, Wadowski PP, Steinlechner B. Different heparin contents in prothrombin complex concentrates may impair blood clotting in outpatients with ventricular assist devices receiving phenprocoumon. J Cardiothorac Vasc Anesth. 2016;30:96–101.

[82] Pabinger I, Tiede A, Kalina U, Knaub S, Germann R, Ostermann H; Beriplex P/N Anticoagulation Reversal Study Group. Impact of infusion speed on the safety and effectiveness of prothrombin complex concentrate: a prospective clinical trial of emergency anticoagulation reversal. Ann Hematol. 2010;89:309–316.

[83] Hirsh J, Anand SS, Halperin JL, Fuster V; American Heart Association. Guide to anticoagulant therapy: heparin: a statement for healthcare professionals from the American Heart Association. Circulation 2001;103:2994–3018.

[84] Ostermann H, Haertel S, Knaub S, Kalina U, Jung K, Pabinger I. Pharmacokinetics of beriplex P/N prothrombin complex concentrate in healthy volunteers. Thromb Haemost. 2007;98:790–797.

[85] Council of Europe. Human prothrombin complex. In: European Pharmacopoeia commission. Human prothrombin complex concentrate. In: European Pharmacopoeia. 8th ed. Strasbourg: Council of Europe, European Directorate for the Quality of Medicines and Healthcare 2013: 2429–2430.

[86] Hellstern P, Beeck H, Fellhauer A, Fischer A, Faller-Stöckl B. Factor VII and activated-factor-VII content of prothrombin complex concentrates. The PCC Study Group. Vox Sang. 1997;73:155–161.

[87] Perry D, Berntorp E, Tait C, Dolan G, Holme PA, Laffan M, Lassila R, Mumford A, Pasi J, Wilde J, Will A, Yee TT. FEIBA prophylaxis in haemophilia patients: a clinical update and treatment recommendations. Haemophilia. 2010;16:80–89.

[88] Furie B, Bouchard BA, Furie BC. Vitamin K-dependent biosynthesis of gamma-carboxyglutamic acid. Blood. 1999,93:1798–1808.

[89] Mann KG, Nesheim ME, Church WR, Haley P, Krishnaswamy S. Surface-dependent reactions of the vitamin K-dependent enzyme complexes. Blood. 1990;76:1–16.

[90] Incampo F, Carrieri C, Galasso R, Scaraggi FA, Di Serio F, Woodhams B, Semeraro N, Colucci M. Effect of warfarin treatment on thrombin activatable fibrinolysis inhibitor (TAFI) activation and TAFI-mediated inhibition of fibrinolysis. J Thromb Haemost. 2013;11:315–324.

[91] D'Angelo A, Della Valle P, Crippa L, Fattorini A, Pattarini E, Viganò D'Angelo S. Relationship between international normalized ratio values, vitamin K-dependent clotting factor levels and in vivo prothrombin activation during the early and steady phases of oral anticoagulant treatment. Haematologica. 2002;87:1074–1080.

[92] Sconce EA, Kamali F. Appraisal of current vitamin K dosing algorithms for the reversal of over-anticoagulation with warfarin: the need for a more tailored dosing regimen. Eur J Haematol. 2006;77:457–462.

[93] Mueck W, Schwers S, Stampfuss J. Rivaroxaban and other novel oral anticoagulants: pharmacokinetics in healthy subjects, specific patient populations and relevance of coagulation monitoring. Thromb J. 2013;11:10.

[94] Dinkelaar J, Patiwael S, Harenberg J, Leyte A, Brinkman HJ. Global coagulation tests: their applicability for measuring direct factor Xa- and thrombin inhibition and reversal of anticoagulation by prothrombin complex concentrate. Clin Chem Lab Med. 2014;52:1615–1623.

[95] Khorsand N, Kooistra HA, van Hest RM, Veeger NJ, Meijer K. A systematic review of prothrombin complex concentrate dosing strategies to reverse vitamin K antagonist therapy. Thromb Res. 2015;135:9–19.

[96] Van Blerk M, Bailleul E, Chatelain B, Demulder A, Devreese K, Douxfils J, Jochmans K, Mullier F, Wijns W, Soumali MR, Coucke W, Vernelen K, Van de Walle P. Influence of dabigatran and rivaroxaban on routine coagulation assays. A nationwide Belgian survey. Thromb Haemost. 2015;113:154–164.

[97] Barrett YC, Wang Z, Frost C, Shenker A. Clinical laboratory measurement of direct factor Xa inhibitors: anti-Xa assay is preferable to prothrombin time assay. Thromb Haemost. 2010;104:1263–1271.

[98] van Aart L, Eijkhout HW, Kamphuis JS, Dam M, Schattenkerk ME, Schouten TJ, Ploeger B, Strengers PF. Individualized dosing regimen for prothrombin complex concentrate more effective than standard treatment in the reversal of oral anticoagulant therapy: an open, prospective randomized controlled trial. Thromb Res. 2006;118:313–320.

[99] Riess HB, Meier-Hellmann A, Motsch J, Elias M, Kursten FW, Dempfle CE. Prothrombin complex concentrate (Octaplex) in patients requiring immediate reversal of oral anticoagulation. Thromb Res. 2007;121:9–16.

[100] Khorsand N, Veeger NJ, van Hest RM, Ypma PF, Heidt J, Meijer K. An observational, prospective, two-cohort comparison of a fixed versus variable dosing strategy of prothrombin complex concentrate to counteract vitamin K antagonists in 240 bleeding emergencies. Haematologica. 2012;97:1501–1506.

[101] Herpers R, van Rossum AP, van Beem RT, Michel WM, Strijbis VJ, Strengers PF, Castel A, Brinkman HJ. INR vs. thrombin generation assays for guiding VKA reversal: a retrospective comparison. Clin Chem Lab Med. 2015;53:1227–1236.

[102] Preston FE, Laidlaw ST, Sampson B, Kitchen S. Rapid reversal of oral anticoagulation with warfarin by a prothrombin complex concentrate (Beriplex): efficacy and safety in 42 patients. Br J Haematol. 2002;116:619–624.

[103] Yasaka M, Sakata T, Naritomi H, Minematsu K. Optimal dose of prothrombin complex concentrate for acute reversal of oral anticoagulation. Thromb Res. 2005;115:455–459.

[104] Pabinger I, Brenner B, Kalina U, Knaub S, Nagy A, Ostermann H; Beriplex P/N Anticoagulation Reversal Study Group. Prothrombin complex concentrate (Beriplex P/N) for emergency anticoagulation reversal: a prospective multinational clinical trial. J Thromb Haemost. 2008;6:622–631.

[105] Altorjay Á, Szabó É, Boda Z, Kramer L, Ngo LY, Engl W, Firth CL, Ahlstrom ER, Gelmont DM, Pabinger I. An international, multicenter, prospective study of a prothrombin complex concentrate, Prothromplex Total®, in anticoagulant reversal. Thromb Res. 2015;135:485–491.

[106] Woo CH, Patel N, Conell C, Rao VA, Faigeles BS, Patel MC, Pombra J, Akins PT, Axelrod YK, Ge IY, Sheridan WF, Flint AC. Rapid Warfarin reversal in the setting of intracranial hemorrhage: a comparison of plasma, recombinant activated factor VII, and prothrombin complex concentrate. World Neurosurg. 2014;81:110–115.

[107] Joseph B, Pandit V, Khalil M, Kulvatunyou N, Aziz H, Tang A, O'Keeffe T, Hays D, Gries L, Lemole M, Friese RS, Rhee P. Use of prothrombin complex concentrate as an adjunct to fresh frozen plasma shortens time to craniotomy in traumatic brain injury patients. Neurosurgery. 2015;76:601–607.

[108] Cartmill M, Dolan G, Byrne JL, Byrne PO. Prothrombin complex concentrate for oral anticoagulant reversal in neurosurgical emergencies. Br J Neurosurg. 2000;14:458–461.

[109] Yanamadala V, Walcott BP, Fecci PE, Rozman P, Kumar JI, Nahed BV, Swearingen B. Reversal of warfarin associated coagulopathy with 4-factor prothrombin complex concentrate in traumatic brain injury and intracranial hemorrhage. J Clin Neurosci. 2014;21:1881–1884.

[110] Milling TJ Jr, Refaai MA, Goldstein JN, Schneider A, Omert L, Harman A, Lee ML, Sarode R. Thromboembolic events after vitamin K antagonist reversal with 4-factor prothrombin complex concentrate: exploratory analyses of two randomized, plasma-controlled studies. Ann Emerg Med. 2016;67:96–105.

[111] Varga C, Al-Touri S, Papadoukakis S, Caplan S, Kahn S, Blostein M. The effectiveness and safety of fixed low-dose prothrombin complex concentrates in patients requiring urgent reversal of warfarin. Transfusion. 2013;53:1451–1458.

[112] Segal JB, Dzik WH; Transfusion Medicine/Hemostasis Clinical Trials Network. Paucity of studies to support that abnormal coagulation test results predict bleeding in the setting of invasive procedures: an evidence-based review. Transfusion. 2005;45:1413–1425.

[113] Sølbeck S, Ostrowski SR, Johansson PI. A review of the clinical utility of INR to monitor and guide administration of prothrombin complex concentrate to orally anticoagulated patients. Thromb J. 2012;10:5.

[114] Brinkman HJ. Global assays and the management of oral anticoagulation. Thromb J. 2015;13:9.

[115] Klein L, Peters J, Miner J, Gorlin J. Evaluation of fixed dose 4-factor prothrombin complex concentrate for emergent warfarin reversal. Am J Emerg Med. 2015;33:1213–1218.

[116] Eerenberg ES, Kamphuisen PW, Sijpkens MK, Meijers JC, Buller HR, Levi M. Reversal of rivaroxaban and dabigatran by prothrombin complex concentrate: a randomized, placebo-controlled, crossover study in healthy subjects. Circulation. 2011;124:1573–1579.

[117] Levi M, Moore KT, Castillejos CF, Kubitza D, Berkowitz SD, Goldhaber SZ, Raghoebar M, Patel MR, Weitz JI, Levy JH. Comparison of three-factor and four-factor prothrombin complex concentrates regarding reversal of the anticoagulant effects of rivaroxaban in healthy volunteers. J Thromb Haemost. 2014;12:1428–1436.

[118] Cheung YW, Barco S, Hutten BA, Meijers JC, Middeldorp S, Coppens M. In vivo increase in thrombin generation by four-factor prothrombin complex concentrate in apixaban-treated healthy volunteers. J Thromb Haemost. 2015;13:1799–1805.

[119] Barco S, Whitney Cheung Y, Coppens M, Hutten BA, Meijers JC, Middeldorp S. In vivo reversal of the anticoagulant effect of rivaroxaban with four-factor prothrombin complex concentrate. Br J Haematol. 2016;172:255–261.

[120] Tanaka KA, Mazzeffi M, Durila M. Role of prothrombin complex concentrate in perioperative coagulation therapy. J Intensive Care. 2014;2:60.

[121] Nowak G. Heparin-induced thrombocytopenia (HIT II) – a drug-associated autoimmune disease. Thromb Haemost. 2009;102:887–891.

[122] Cappabianca G, Mariscalco G, Biancari F, Maselli D, Papesso F, Cottini M, Crosta S, Banescu S, Ahmed AB, Beghi C. Safety and efficacy of prothrombin complex concentrate as first-line treatment in bleeding after cardiac surgery. Crit Care. 2016;20:5.

[123] Lind SE, Callas PW, Golden EA, Joyner KA Jr, Ortel TL. Plasma levels of factors II, VII and X and their relationship to the international normalized ratio during chronic warfarin therapy. Blood Coagul Fibrinolysis. 1997;8:48–53.

[124] Dinkelaar J, Molenaar PJ, Ninivaggi M, de Laat B, Brinkman HJ, Leyte A. In vitro assessment, using thrombin generation, of the applicability of prothrombin complex concentrate as an antidote for Rivaroxaban. J Thromb Haemost. 2013;11:1111–1118.

Chapter 6

Non-Vitamin K Antagonist Oral Anticoagulants in Atrial Fibrillation: Pharmacology and Phase III Clinical Trials

Keval K. Patel, Ali A. Mehdirad and Richard Lee

Additional information is available at the end of the chapter

http://dx.doi.org/10.5772/64440

Abstract

Atrial fibrillation (AF) is a very common clinically significant arrhythmia noted in clinical practice. Its incidence increases with age and along with advanced age, other risk factors such hypertension, vascular disease, heart failure, diabetes, prior stroke and female sex determine the associated stroke risk with AF. For over 40 years warfarin has been the drug of choice used to reduce this stroke risk associated with AF. However, the narrow therapeutic range, dietary restrictions, and chronic monitoring with warfarin led to the development of novel oral anticoagulants (NOACs) such as dabigatran, rivaroxaban, apixaban, and edoxaban. The purpose of this chapter is to elucidate pharmacology and the clinical performance of these NOACs in the setting of non-valvular atrial fibrillation (NVAF).

Keywords: novel oral anticoagulants, non-valvular atrial fibrillation, dabigatran, rivaroxaban, apixaban, edoxaban, stroke prevention, atrial fibrilation

1. Introduction

Atrial fibrillation (AF) is one of the most common arrhythmias in clinical practice affecting approximately 2.3 million people in the United States and 4.5 million people in Europe. The incidence increases with age and the prevalence being 9% between the ages of 80 and 90 [1]. Other risk factors include hypertension, coronary artery disease, chronic obstructive pulmonary disease, valvular heart diseases or surgeries, hyperthyroidism and chronic alcoholism. The mortality rate in AF is twice that of age-matched individuals in normal sinus rhythm, and stroke risk is increased approximately fivefold in patients with non-valvular atrial fibrillation (NVAF) [2].

Over the last five decades, vitamin K antagonists (VKAs) such as warfarin have been the only oral anticoagulants available for use as a long-term treatment to prevent strokes in patients with AF. Aspirin (ASA) may be used for patients with NVAF who cannot take warfarin for one reason or another, but ASA is much less effective than warfarin and is therefore recommended only for NVAF patients at low risk of stroke (CHA2DS2-VASc score of 0 or 1) in the American College of Chest Physicians (ACCP) guidelines [2–4]. The CHA2DS2-VASc score is an improvement on the CHADS2 score which has been widely used in clinical practice to risk stratify patients with NVAF for stroke. The CHA2DS2-VASc added three risk factors, namely age 65–74, female sex, and history of vascular disease [5]. However, the clinical trials for novel oral anticoagulants (NOACs) were conducted prior to widespread implementation of the CHA2DS2-VASc score, and thus, the risk stratification used in the trials is CHADS2.

Several historical placebo-controlled trials in subjects with AF were conducted with warfarin between 1989 and 1999. A meta-analysis of these historical trials using a fixed effects model showed that the relative risk reduction of stroke by warfarin was 62% (95% CI: 0.48, 0.72) with an absolute risk reduction of 2.7% for primary prevention and 8.4% for secondary prevention per year [2].

Although warfarin has been proven to be highly effective in preventing strokes, there have been multiple issues such as periodic monitoring, dietary restrictions, medication restrictions or interactions, and concerns for bleeding which render many patients with NVAF ineligible to receive warfarin therapy. For example, a registry of patients discharged from hospital revealed that only 54% of eligible AF patients received warfarin [6]. Likewise, surveys have indicated that many patients with AF cannot or will not take warfarin. Only 10% of patients with known AF who presented with an acute ischemic stroke had a therapeutic INR on admission, and even in those AF patients with a prior history of stroke or transient ischemic attack (TIA), only 18% had a therapeutic INR on admission [7]. Furthermore, studies show that the risk of intracranial hemorrhage was more than twice that of patients taking aspirin [2]. Thus, there was a need to develop an anticoagulant that would have similar or better efficacy as compared with warfarin along with better safety and more convenient management. Dabigatran, rivaroxaban, apixaban, and edoxaban have been approved over the past five years to satisfy this need.

2. Pharmacology

2.1. Mechanism of action

Dabigatran acts as a competitive reversible direct inhibitor of thrombin thereby preventing the thrombin-dependent conversion of fibrinogen to fibrin in the coagulation cascade. Rivaroxaban, apixaban, and edoxaban are direct competitive inhibitors of factor Xa, thereby inhibiting the formation of thrombin from prothrombin and downstream formation of fibrin from

http://dx.doi.org/10.5772/64440

fibrinogen. And since factor Xa is located at the top of the final common coagulation pathway, rivaroxaban, apixaban, and edoxaban can affect both the intrinsic and extrinsic coagulation cascades. These target coagulation factors and other pharmacological parameters for each drug are summarized in **Table 1**.

Characteristic	Dabigatran	Rivaroxaban	Apixaban	Edoxaban
Target	Factor IIa	Factor Xa	Factor Xa	Factor Xa
Molecular weight (Dal)	724	436	460	738
Ki (nmol/l)	4.6	0.4	0.08	0.56
Concentration to double PT (μmol/l)	0.8	0.23	0.08	0.26
Concentration to double PTT (μmol/l)	0.23	0.69	7.4	0.51
Reversible binding	Yes	Yes	Yes	Yes
Reversal of antithrombotic effect	Specific antidote: Idarucizumab May consider PCC, APCC, rFVIIa	May consider PCC, APCC, rFVIIa	May consider PCC, APCC, rFVIIa	May consider PCC, APCC, rFVIIa
Half-life (h)	12–17	5–9	12	10–14
Cmax (h)	1	2–4	3–4	1–2
Volume of distribution (l)	50–70	~50	21	107
Protein binding	35%	92–95%	87%	55%
Renal excretion	80%	66%	27%	50%
Accumulation	None	None	None	None
Age effect	None	None	Yes§	None
Sex effect	None	None	None	None
Body weight effect	None	None	Yes	Yes
Effect of food	Yes*	Yes	None	None
Primary hepatic clearance pathway	No	CYP3A4	CYP3A4	No
Pregnancy category	C	C	B	C

* Increases Cmax to 2 h but does not affect bioavailability.
§ Dosage reduction recommended if two of the following three risk factors present: body weight <60 kg, age >80 years or serum creatinine >1.5 mg/dl.

Table 1. Pharmacokinetics and pharmacodynamics.

2.2. Absorption

Dabigatran itself is not absorbed via the oral route; however, its prodrug dabigatran etexilate is rapidly absorbed (bioavailability 3–7%) via the oral route and is converted to the active ingredient by esterase-mediated hydrolysis in the liver. The absorption increases significantly when the capsules are broken, and thus, the capsules should not be broken or chewed or opened prior to administration. Additionally, when taken concomitantly with highly fatty food, the time to maximal concentration (Cmax) increases from 1 to 2 h but the bioavailability is not affected [8]. Rivaroxaban is rapidly absorbed in the proximal intestine with maximum concentrations (Cmax) appearing 2–4 h after tablet intake with the absolute bioavailability of 80% for the 10 mg dose and 66% for the 20 mg dose. The bioavailability is decreased when the drug is absorbed in the distal intestine or ascending colon [9]. This is an important consideration for patients with gastric bypass or other GI conditions that cause rapid transit. When taken with food, both the Cmax and the bioavailability of rivaroxaban (for both 15 and 20 mg doses) increases by 39 and 76%, respectively [9]. Thus, it is recommended that rivaroxaban be taken with a large meal (ideally dinner) and not a light meal in order to slow down the transit time.

Unlike the first two, apixaban is absorbed throughout the gastrointestinal tract, and therefore, the drug displays a prolonged absorption which is not affected by food intake. The absolute bioavailability of apixaban is 50% for doses up to 10 mg with a Cmax of 3–4 h. The distal small bowel and ascending colon account for 55% of the absorption of apixaban. Thereby, making it a better choice for patients with gastric bypass or other gastrointestinal conditions which lead to rapid transit, whereas in patients with colectomies or Crohn's disease, etc., apixaban's absorption may be altered and the drug may not be as readily available.

Edoxaban is also absorbed predominantly by the upper gastrointestinal tract with Cmax of 1–2 h and bioavailability of 62%. The colon only accounts for 12% of absorption, thereby rendering the absorption of the drug susceptible to conditions that cause rapid transit, similar to rivaroxaban [10]. However unlike rivaroxaban, the absorption of edoxaban is not significantly affected by food intake.

2.3. P-glycoprotein transporter, cytochrome P-450 (CYP) enzymes, and drug interactions

The pro-drug dabigatran etexilate is a substrate for the efflux transporter P-glycoprotein (p-GP) transporter. And even though it neither induces nor inhibits p-GP, potential co-administration of other drugs that inhibit or induce P-GP can affect its bioavailability. The pharmacokinetics of dabigatran were not altered by another p-GP substrate digoxin, but an inhibitor like pantoprazole decreased the bioavailability by 30% [11]. Since H2 blocker ranitidine has no effect on the p-GP transporter, there was no effect on the area under the curve (AUC) when dabigatran was co-administered. For other p-GP inhibitors such as dronedarone or systemic ketoconazole, dosage adjustment was required in patients with reduced creatinine clearance (30–50 ml/min) [8]. Other p-GP inhibitors such as amiodarone and verapamil only modestly increased plasma concentrations (13 and 20%, respectively), and dose adjustment is not required for these medications [11]. On the other hand, potent p-GP inducers such as such as rifampin significantly reduced the AUC and Cmax of dabigatran and concomitant use should therefore be avoided. Dabigatran is neither a substrate, nor an inducer or inhibitor of CYP enzymes [8].

Rivaroxaban is a substrate for p-GP transporter, CYP3A4/5 enzymes, and other transporters such as ATP-binding cassette G2 [9]. Approximately 51% of orally administered rivaroxaban is metabolized by the CYP enzymes 3A4 and 3A5. Thus, inhibition or induction of these proteins can lead to changes in the bioavailability of the drug. When studied with rifampin or phenytoin (p-GP and strong CYP3A4 inducers), the exposure to rivaroxaban decreased by 50%. Similarly, other combined strong p-GP, CYP3A4 inducers such as carbamazepine, phenytoin, rifampin, and St. John's wort should be avoided in patients taking rivaroxaban. For drugs that are combined p-GP and CYP3A4 inhibitors (ketoconazole, ritonavir, clarithromycin, and erythromycin) or a moderate CYP3A4 inhibitor (fluconazole), studies showed increases in rivaroxaban exposure [9]. A dosage adjustment to 15 mg is required when taking these medications concomitantly in patients with decreased creatinine clearance (CrCl 15–50 ml/min). Additionally, rivaroxaban also has a low inhibitory effect on the p-GP transporter. Regardless, there were no significant interactions with 7.5 mg single dose of midazolam (substrate of CYP3A4), 0.375 mg once-daily dose of digoxin (substrate of p-GP), and 20 mg once-daily dose of atorvastatin (substrate of CYP3A4 and p-GP) in healthy volunteers [12]. This is interesting because although neither dabigatran nor rivaroxaban has significant interactions with digoxin, rivaroxaban may be a better choice for patients with severe ischemic cardiomyopathy and NVAF because of an increased incidence of myocardial infarctions seen with dabigatran (discussed later).

Like dabigatran, apixaban is also a substrate for p-GP efflux transporter but unlike dabigatran, inhibition of p-GP transporter by itself does not affect the bioavailability. The drug is also metabolized by CYP3A4 and co-administration with drugs that are strong inducers and inhibitors for both p-GP and CYP3A4 increases the exposure to apixaban and raises the risk of bleeding. Rifampin, carbamazepine, phenytoin, and St. John's wort are strong combined inducers of p-GP and CYP34A and thus concomitant use should be avoided due to reduced exposure to apixaban. Ketoconazole, itraconazole, ritonavir, clarithromycin are strong dual inhibitors of p-GP and CYP3A4 and thus can increase exposure to apixaban [13]. Dose adjustment to 2.5 mg is recommended when apixaban is taken concomitantly with these medications. If the patient is already on the reduced dose (2.5 mg) of apixaban for other reasons, concomitant use of these medications is contraindicated [13]. Apixaban does not inhibit or induce p-GP and its potential to inhibit or induce CYP enzymes is minimal and as such the ability of apixaban to alter the exposure of co-administered drugs that are metabolites for these enzymes is minimal.

Unlike rivaroxaban and apixaban, CYP enzymes only account for 4% of the exposure to edoxaban. However, the intestinal p-GP transporter plays a significant role in clearance of the drug and thus inhibition of the transporter leads to increased exposure. Clinical interaction studies showed exposure to edoxaban increased by 87, 77, 53, 85, 73, 40, and 85% when used concomitantly with ketoconazole, quinidine, verapamil, erythromycin, cyclosporine, amiodarone, and dronedarone, respectively [10]. Subsequently in ENGAGE trial, the edoxaban was halved to 30 mg in patients who were taking verapamil, quinidine, or dronedarone [14]. And in the HOKUSAI VTE study, the dose was reduced for patients taking verapamil, quinidine, azithromycin, clarithromycin, erythromycin, itraconazole, or ketoconazole [15]. The use of edoxaban should be avoided when taking a potent p-GP inducer like rifampin, phenytoin, carbamazepine, and St. John's wort [16].

2.4. Elimination

In the phases II and III of the RE-LY trial, dabigatran was administered in oral, intramuscular, and intravenous formulations. After oral administration of radiolabeled dabigatran, 82.6–88.6% of radioactivity was recovered in the feces and 7% was recovered in the urine, the remaining was attributed to incomplete absorption of dabigatran. Renal clearance of intravenous dabigatran was approximately 80%. After infusion, the total clearance of dabigatran was found to be 92–141 ml/min, and the renal clearance was 81–106 ml/min showing that dabigatran is almost exclusively excreted via glomerular filtration and there was no secretion or reabsorption further down the tubule [7, 13]. The terminal half-life was 12–17 h in healthy individuals. The half-life was confounded by renal impairment and was increased to 15, 18, and 27.2 h, respectively, in mild (50–80 ml/min), moderate (30–50 ml/min), and severe (15–30) renal insufficiency. The total exposure (or AUC) also increased by approximately 1.5-, 3.2-, and 6.3-fold in mild, moderate, and severe renal impairment, respectively, when compared to normal renal function. It is thus recommended that the dose of dabigatran for atrial fibrillation be halved to 75 mg when the creatinine clearance (CrCl) is between 15 and 30 ml/min for and the use of dabigatran should be avoided in patients with CrCl less than 15 ml/min or those on dialysis [8]. Administration of dabigatran in patients with moderate (Child-Pugh class B) liver impairment showed large inter-subject variability, but no evidence of a consistent change in exposure or pharmacodynamics because the primary elimination pathway for dabigatran is via the kidneys [8].

Off the orally administered radiolabeled rivaroxaban, 66% was recovered in the urine (36% unchanged) and 28% was recovered in the feces (7%). The renal excretion of rivaroxaban is primarily driven by active tubular secretion and secondarily by glomerular filtration in a 5:1 ratio. The terminal half-life is 5–9 h in healthy young individuals [9, 12]. Like dabigatran, the exposure to rivaroxaban also increases by 44% for mild, 52% for moderate, and 66% for severe renal impairment. As such, it is recommended that the dose of rivaroxaban for stroke prevention in NVAF be reduced to 15 mg orally with dinner in patients with moderate-to-severe renal impairment (CrCl 15–50 ml/min) due to increased exposure and rivaroxaban should be avoided in patients with CrCl <15 ml/min or those on dialysis. Rivaroxaban was not studied in patients with severe (Child-Pugh class C) hepatic impairment, and exposure to rivaroxaban increased by 15 and 127% in patients with Child-Pugh class A and B hepatic impairment [9].

Unlike dabigatran and rivaroxaban, apixaban is excreted in both urine and feces. Renal excretion accounts for 27% of total clearance and biliary, and direct intestinal excretion accounts towards the fecal elimination of apixaban. The terminal half-life is 12 h, and the exposure is not significantly affected (<1.5× normal) for any level of renal impairment including end-stage renal disease. Thus, no dosing adjustment is recommended kidney disease alone. However, a dosage reduction of apixaban to 2.5 mg is recommended in patients that meet another one of the following two risk factors: age >80 years or body weight <60 kg [13]. However, it should be noted that patients with end-stage renal disease (CrCl <15 ml/min) were not studied in the clinical efficacy and safety trials [16]. The recommendation for no dosage adjustment is based on pharmacokinetic data showing a modest 17% increase in apixaban exposure in patients receiving hemodialysis with an elimination via dialysis of 18 ml/min reducing exposure of the drug by 14% postdialysis as compared to off dialysis period. Similarly, in patients with mild (Child-Pugh A) and moderate (Child-Pugh B) hepatic impairment, the area under the curve or exposure did not change significantly as compared to normal individuals and no dose adjustment is necessary in patients with Child-Pugh class A hepatic impairment. However, since patients who have Child-Pugh class B hepatic impairment may have intrinsic coagulation abnormalities, a recommendation on dosing cannot be made due to limited clinical experience. Like the others, use of apixaban is not recommended in patients with severe (Child-Pugh class C) hepatic impairment [13].

Edoxaban is excreted as unchanged drug in the urine with renal clearance accounting for 50% of total clearance. Metabolism as well as biliary and intestinal excretion accounts for the remaining clearance. The terminal half-life is 10–14 h. In a pharmacokinetic study, the total systemic exposure to edoxaban increased by 32, 74, and 72% in patients with mild (50–80 ml/min), moderate (30–50 ml/min), severe (15–30 ml/min) renal impairment, and by 93% in patients receiving dialysis. Thus, a reduction in dose to 30 mg daily is recommended in patients with CrCl 15–50 ml/min for stroke prevention in non-valvular atrial fibrillation [10, 16]. Interestingly, the incidence of stroke was higher in patients receiving edoxaban who had a CrCl >95 ml/min as compared to warfarin in the clinical trial and the use of edoxaban is not recommended in these patients [10, 14]. There were no significant differences for edoxaban in patients with mild or moderate (Child-Pugh class A or B) hepatic impairment. A dose adjustment is not necessary for Class A patients; however, once again due to the intrinsic coagulation abnormalities in patients with class B hepatic impairment, the use of edoxaban is not recommended [16].

2.5. Special populations

The pharmacokinetics and pharmacodynamics of both dabigatran and rivaroxaban are not affected by age, gender, or body weight. There is no effect of ethnicity on the pharmacology of dabigatran either, but rivaroxaban did have 20–40% higher exposure in patients of Japanese ethnicity as compared to other ethnicities including Chinese [9]. This exposure was reduced when it was corrected for body weight, but further studies may be required to assess clinical implications to the use of rivaroxaban in the Japanese population specifically. Although individually aged over 80 years and body weight <60 kg only modestly increased the exposure to apixaban (<1.5× normal individuals), the combination of the two risk factors was deemed to have a significant increase in the exposure of the drug. Thus, a reduced dose of 2.5 mg was used in ARISTOTLE for patients who had two of the following three risk factors: age older than 80 years, body weight <60 kg, and creatinine >1.5 mg/dl [13, 17]. Age is not a risk factor for increased exposure of edoxaban but a phase II open-label study done in Japan revealed that patients with total body weight <60 kg had double the bleeding risk as compared to patients with total body weight >60 kg. Thus, in the phase III clinical trial, the dose of edoxaban was reduced to 30 mg daily in patients with total body weight <60 kg [14, 16].

Dabigatran, rivaroxaban, and edoxaban are all under category C for pregnancy. Animal studies showed increased maternal bleeding and increased fetal mortality with all three drugs. There was decreased fetal implantation with dabigatran, and increased post-implantation loss, and decreased fetal weight with rivaroxaban and edoxaban [8, 9, 16]. Additionally, there was decrease in gall bladder size or absence of the organ with the use of edoxaban in animal studies. Ten pregnancies were reported during the HOKUSAI VTE study, from which there were four full-term births, two preterm births, one spontaneous abortion in the first trimester, and three elective terminations during the study [15, 16]. In comparison, animal studies with apixaban did not cause an increase in fetal toxicity, malformations, or mortality. There was an increase in the rate of maternal bleeding at the rate of 19, 4, and 1 times, respectively, for mice, rats, and rabbits with apixaban. As a result, the use of apixaban is under category B for pregnancy [13]. None of the NOACs are recommended for mothers who are breastfeeding, and the use of these drugs has not been studied in the pediatric population.

3. Clinical trials

3.1. Trial designs

The Randomized Evaluation of Long-term Anticoagulation Therapy (RE-LY) trial was designed as a non-inferiority trial to compare dabigatran to warfarin in 18, 113 patients from 951 clinical centers in 44 countries. Two doses of dabigatran; 110 and 150 mg were administered in a double-blinded fashion [18]. We will discuss the data for the 150 mg dose of dabigatran as FDA approval was only obtained for 150 and 75 mg (not studied) doses. The warfarin arm was not blinded because the patients taking it needed regular follow-ups for INR control. The semi-blinded design of RE-LY could leave the trial open to reporter bias. Thus, the authors of the trial tried to minimize this bias by assigning two independent investigators who were unaware of the treatment assignments, to adjudicate each event. In addition, all hospital records were reviewed to ensure that all events were detected and correctly documented [18]. In contrast, the other three trials were designed in a double-blinded double dummy randomized fashion to avoid reporter bias.

The Rivaroxaban Once-Daily Oral Direct Factor Xa Inhibition Compared with Vitamin K Antagonism for Prevention of Stroke and Embolism Trial in Atrial Fibrillation (ROCKET-AF) trial studied Warfarin in comparison with 20 mg of rivaroxaban in 14,264 patients from 1178 centers in 45 countries [19]. Similarly, the apixaban for Reduction in Stroke and Other Thromboembolic Events in Atrial Fibrillation (ARISTOTLE) study enrolled 18,201 patients at 1034 sites in 39 countries and Effective Anticoagulation with Factor Xa Next Generation in Atrial Fibrillation-Thrombolysis in Myocardial Infarction 48 (ENGAGE AF-TIMI 48) enrolled 21,105 patients from 1393 centers in 46 countries to study apixaban 5 mg and edoxaban 60 mg to warfarin, respectively [14, 17].

Lower doses of NOACs were studied in ROCKET, ARISTOTLE, and ENGAGE. Rivaroxaban 15 mg was used for patients with creatinine clearance 15–50 ml/min [19]. For ARISTOTLE,

http://dx.doi.org/10.5772/64440

apixaban dose was reduced to 2.5 mg twice daily if the patient had two of the following three risk factors for increased bleeding: age ≥80 years, body weight ≤60 kg, or a serum creatinine level ≥1.5 mg per deciliter [17]. In ENGAGE, randomization was done in 1:1:1 fashion for warfarin, edoxaban 60 mg, and edoxaban 30 mg. The doses of edoxaban were further halved to 30 and 15 mg for patients who either had a creatinine clearance 30–50 ml/min or body weight ≤60 kg thereby allowing a range of doses from 15 to 60 mg to be used in the study [14]. However, the results of the study were more promising from the 60 mg dose with reduction to 30 mg for specific patients leading to FDA approval. Thus, for the scope of this chapter, only the results pertaining edoxaban 60 mg daily dose will be discussed.

Additionally, ROCKET-AF used both intention-to-treat and on-treatment analyses, and the outcomes listed as number of events per 100 patient-years (instead of percent per year) [19]. To facilitate comparisons between trials, only the intention-to-treat analyses are reported in this chapter. Similarly, ENGAGE also had a prespecified intention-to-treat analysis to assess superiority to warfarin which was not statistically significant and thus will not be discussed for the purposes of this chapter.

3.2. Patient populations

All four trials used similar criteria for enrolling and following patients with subtle differences as listed in **Table 2**. However, these subtle differences may affect decision-making in different clinical scenarios. For example, only ENGAGE included patients with prior bioprosthetic valve or valve repair and as such edoxaban may be the preferred agent for stroke prevention in these patients. Similarly, for newly diagnosed strokes, ARISTOTLE excluded patients with strokes within 7 days of randomization. RE-LY, ROCKET, and ENGAGE excluded patients with strokes within 6, 3, and 1 month, respectively. RE-LY and ROCKET also excluded patients with transient ischemic attack (TIA) within 14 days and thus if a patient has had a stroke more than 7 days prior to and within 1 month of planned anticoagulation, apixaban may be the preferred agent. ARISTOTLE also included patients with creatinine clearance less than 30 ml/min and had the most patients in this category. As such in the absence of other risk factors for bleeding and increased exposure to apixaban, the use of apixaban would be preferred in these patients.

Another important consideration is the CHADS2 score used in the trial, because higher scores are associated with incrementally higher risk of stroke. Both ROCKET and ENGAGE required a minimum $CHADS_2$ score of 2 to be included in the trial. Additionally, ROCKET also permitted patients with lower left ventricular ejection fractions, thus enrolling a higher risk patient population than RE-LY and ARISTOTLE. Roughly one-third of patients in RE-LY and ARISTOTLE had $CHADS_2$ scores of 0 or 1, resulting in an overall 1% lower absolute risk of stroke in those patients as compared to those enrolled in ROCKET or ENGAGE. Even though the $CHADS_2$ score was evenly distributed between the drug and warfarin groups were evenly distributed in both trials, the overall incidence of primary outcome could be overestimated for the ROCKET and ENGAGE trials.

Characteristic	RE-LY	ROCKET	ARISTOTLE	ENGAGE
Drug	Dabigatran	Rivaroxaban	Apixaban	Edoxaban
Dosing	150 mg BID (75 mg)	20 mg daily (15 mg)	5 mg BID (2.5 mg)	60 mg daily (30 mg)
Total population (N)	18,113	14,266	18,206	21,105
Design	PROBE	Double blinded	Double blinded	Double blinded
Primary efficacy endpoint	Stroke or systemic embolism	Stroke or systemic embolism	Stroke or systemic embolism	Stroke or systemic embolism
Primary safety endpoint	Major bleeding	Major bleeding or clinically relevant non-major Bleeding	Major bleeding	Major bleeding
VKA naïve	50%	38%	43%	41%
Mean TTR for INR during study	64	55	62	68
Inclusion criteria				
AF criteria	AF at screening or within 6 months	AF recorded in 30 days prior to randomization and within 1 year	2 episodes of AF or flutter recorded 2 weeks apart within 1 year	AF recorded within 1 year
LVEF	40% or less	35% or less	40% or less	NA
Exclusion criteria				
Valve disease	Hemodynamically significant or prosthetic	Hemodynamically significant or prosthetic	Moderate-severe mitral stenosis or prosthetic	Moderate-severe mitral stenosis or mechanical§
Stroke	Severe w/in 6 months or TIA w/in 14 days	Severe w/in 3 months or TIA w/in 14 days	Stroke w/in 7days	Stroke w/in 30 days
Bleeding	Surgery w/in 30 days, GI bleed w/in 12 months, any intracranial bleed, severe hypertension	Surgery w/in 30 days, GI bleed w/in 6mo, active internal bleeding, any intracranial bleed, dual antiplatelet therapy, severe hypertension, platelet ≤90,000	Any intracranial bleed, dual antiplatelet therapy, severe hypertension	High risk for bleeding, dual antiplatelet therapy
Patient demographics				
Age (yrs)	71	71	70	72

http://dx.doi.org/10.5772/64440

Characteristic	RE-LY	ROCKET	ARISTOTLE	ENGAGE
Male gender (%)	63.2	60.3	64.5	61.9
Type of atrial fibrillation (%)				
Paroxysmal	32.6	17.5	15.1	25.4
Persistent/ permanent	67.4	82.5	84.9	74.6
$CHADS_2$score (%)				
I	32.2	0	34	0
II	35.2	13	35.8	46.8
III–VI	32.6	87	30.2	53.2
Comorbidities (%)				
Hypertension	78.9	74	87.3	93.6
Previous TIA	20.3	54.9	19.2	28.3
Diabetes	23.1	40.4	25	36.2
Heart failure	31.8	62.6	35.5	57.5
Prior MI, CAD, CABG	28	17.3	14.5	33.3
Medications (%)				
ACE or ARB	66.7	55.1	70.9	65.9
Beta-blockers	63.7	65.1	63.6	66.3
Digoxin	28.7	38.8	32	30
Amiodarone	10.9	NA	11.1	11.8
Statins	43.9	42.9	45	47.8
Gastric antacids	17.9*	NA	18.5	NA
NSAIDS	1.4	NA	8.2	1.1
Aspirin	38.7	36.3	31.3	29.3
Thienopyridine	5.5	NA	1.9	2.3
Creatinine clearance (%)				
>80 ml/min	32	32.2	41.2	37.2
>50–80 ml/min	47.4	46.7	41.9	43
>30–50 ml/min	19.7	21.1	15	18.4
<30 ml/min	0.005	NA	1.5	0.76

* Total of proton pump inhibitors 13.9% and H_2 antagonists 4%.
§ Bioprosthetic valves or valve repair patients were included.

Table 2. Study design and patient demographics.

3.3. INR control

INR control is probably the most important factor in determining the non-inferiority of NOACs. All trials used the Rosendaal method of total time in therapeutic range (TTR, reflecting the percent of time the patient had an INR between 2 and 3) [20]. Overall, the TTR was 64% in the RE-LY trial, 55% in ROCKET, 62% for ARISTOTLE, and 68% for ENGAGE. These numbers clearly reflect that ROCKET had the least robust INR control in the warfarin arm leading to significant criticism of the trial.

Although these data were not analyzed further in the primary publications, the heterogeneity of INR management in the other trials appeared to impact clinical outcomes. In RE-LY, the INR control in east and South-East Asia was worse than centers in Europe and North America. The hazard ratio for major bleeding with dabigatran 150 mg was 1.24 (p = 0.03) when the TTR was 68% or more [11]. Additionally, higher rates of both thromboembolic events and major bleeds were seen with warfarin in centers with TTR <57%, even after adjusting for multiple other potential confounding variables [21]. The inadequacy of INR control in Asia may explain the more robust performance of dabigatran in those centers. Dabigatran 150 mg also performed better than warfarin for a composite of stroke, systemic embolism, pulmonary embolism, myocardial infarction, and cardiovascular death with a hazard ratio of 0.64 for TTR <57.1 and hazard ratio of 1.19 for TTR 72.6 (p = 0.006). This trend was mirrored in the mortality rate where dabigatran had an advantage at the centers with poor INR control (HR 0.67 vs 1.08, p = 0.052) [21].

Similar to dabigatran, edoxaban also had lower efficacy in patients with higher TTR. The hazard ratio for edoxaban 60 mg vs warfarin in TTR <57.7 was 0.8 compared to hazard ratio of 1.07 for patients with TTR >73.9. TTR [10]. A different issue was noted in ROCKET-AF, the TTR was low for the trial overall trial, and the resultant bleeding risks were equivalent between rivaroxaban and warfarin. However, the centers in the USA where TTR was around 64%, patients taking rivaroxaban suffered 2.5–3.7 more bleeds per stroke prevented as compared to those taking warfarin [12]. Overall in patients with excellent INR control, warfarin may still be the drug of choice for stroke prevention in atrial fibrillation.

3.4. Results and discussion

The primary outcome in all four trials was stroke or systemic embolism, and the primary safety endpoint was major bleeding (RE-LY, ARISTOTLE, and ENGAGE), or combined major and clinically important non-major bleeding events (ROCKET). As illustrated in **Table 3**, patients randomized to the 150 mg dose of dabigatran in RE-LY had a reduction in the primary outcome, experienced fewer ischemic as well as hemorrhagic strokes, and had a strong trend toward lower all-cause mortality in spite of experiencing higher rates of myocardial infarction [18]. This trend for higher myocardial infarction leads to several meta-analyses which showed approximately 30–40% increase in the rates of myocardial infarction with the use of dabigatran as compared to control arms including enoxaparin, placebo, and warfarin [22, 23]. However, in a post market analysis of 134,000 Medicare patients over 65 years of age done by the FDA did not show any difference between the incidence of myocardial infarction between Dabigatran (15.7 per 1000 person years) and warfarin (16.9 per 1000 person years, p 0.92) [24]. None

http://dx.doi.org/10.5772/64440

Clinical outcome	RE-LY				ROCKET				ARISTOTLE				ENGAGE			
	Dabigatran 150 mg BID, %/y	**Warfarin %/y**	**Hazard ratio**	**p value**	**Rivaroxaban 20 mg QD, %/y**	**Warfarin %/y**	**Hazard ratio**	**p value**	**Apixaban 5 mg BID, %/y**	**Warfarin %/y**	**Hazard Ratio**	**p value**	**Edoxaban high dose %/y**	**Warfarin %/y**	**Hazard Ratio**	**p value**
Stroke or SAE	1.11	1.69	0.66	<0.001	2.1	2.4	0.88	<0.001	1.27	1.6	0.79	0.01	1.18	1.5	0.79	<0.001
Stroke	1.01	1.57	0.64	<0.001	1.65	1.96	0.85	0.092	1.19	1.51	0.79	0.01	0.26	0.47	0.54	<0.001
Ischemic	0.92	1.2	0.76	0.03	1.34	1.42	0.94	0.581	0.97	1.05	0.92	0.42	1.25	1.25	1	0.97
Hemorrhagic	26.1	0.38	0.26	<0.001	0.26	0.44	0.59	0.024	0.24	0.47	0.51	<0.001	0.26	0.47	0.54	<0.001
Disabling	0.66	1	0.66	0.005	0.39	0.5	0.77	0.188	0.5	0.71	0.71	0.94	0.28	0.3	0.94	0.75
Non-disabling	0.37	0.58	0.62	0.01	0.79	0.77	1.03	0.863					0.81	1.01	0.8	0.044
Myocardial infarction	0.74	0.53	1.38	0.048	0.91	1.12	0.81	0.121	0.53	0.61	0.88	0.37	0.7	0.75	0.94	0.6
Death from vascular cause	2.28	2.69	0.85	0.04	1.53	1.71	0.89	0.289								
All-cause mortality	3.64	4.13	0.88	0.051	1.87	2.21	0.85	0.073	3.52	3.94	0.89	0.047	3.8	4.35	0.87	0.006
Major bleeds	3.11	3.36	0.93	0.3	3.6	3.4	1.04	0.58	2.13	3.09	0.69	<0.001	2.75	3.43	0.8	<0.001
Intracranial bleeds	0.3	0.74	0.4	<0.001	0.5	0.7	0.67	0.02	0.33	0.8	0.42	<0.001	0.38	0.85	0.47	<0.001
GI bleeds	1.51	1.02	1.5	<0.001	3.15*	2.16*		<0.001	0.76	0.86	0.89	0.37	1.51	1.23	1.23	0.03

* Gastrointestinal bleeds in ROCKET-AF were reported as percentages and no Hazard ratio was reported, whereas all other outcomes in this trial were reported as number per 100 patient-years.

Table 3. Efficacy outcomes.

of the other NOAC had any signal towards myocardial infarction in their respective trials and the choice of using an alternative agent to dabigatran in the setting of known coronary artery disease should be individualized based on the clinical setting and physician discretion. There was no difference in overall major bleeding, where a significant reduction in intracranial hemorrhage was offset by a significantly higher rate of gastrointestinal bleeding.

For the intention-to-treat analyses in ROCKET-AF, rivaroxaban was noted to be non-inferior (but not superior) to warfarin in reducing the primary endpoint [19]. The reduction in ischemic stroke was not statistically significant as compared to the warfarin group and the outcomes were driven by a significant reduction in hemorrhagic stroke by rivaroxaban which may be reflective of the poor INR control in the trial. There was a trend toward reducing all-cause mortality in ROCKET, and like RE-LY, an equivalent bleeding endpoint was driven by a significant reduction of intracranial hemorrhage in the setting higher rates of gastrointestinal bleeds. In comparison, apixaban was the only drug to show statistically significant reduction in primary outcome compared to warfarin in both non-inferiority and superiority analyses. And, like the other trials, the reduction in the primary outcome was driven by a significant reduction of hemorrhagic strokes [17]. ENGAGE did show non-inferiority to warfarin in the reduction of primary outcomes, but in the prespecified superiority analysis, the difference was not statistically significant [14]. Unlike the prior studies of dabigatran and rivaroxaban, both ARISTOTLE and ENGAGE demonstrated a statistically significant reduction in all-cause mortality and major bleeding with the study drugs in comparison to warfarin [14, 17]. However, only apixaban showed no significant increase in gastrointestinal bleeding among all NOACs and it should be considered as the agent of choice in patients with prior (or at high risk for) gastrointestinal bleeding.

4. Conclusion

The approval of NOACs for stroke prevention in patients with NVAF has ushered a new era in this field with a multitude of options available for practitioners. Warfarin still may be the drug of choice in several clinical situations such as compliant patients with good INR control or those with valvular heart disease, etc. However, patient preference and the ease of use have made NOACs the preferred initial agent for stroke prevention in patients with NVAF. The subtle differences between the NOACs described throughout this chapter are aimed at providing an improved understanding of the intricacies with which these medications perform in the human body and thereby help guide decision-making.

5. Conflicts of interest and source of funding

No grant or other financial support was used for writing this chapter. Dr. Mehdirad has been a speaker for Apixaban.

Author details

Keval K. Patel*, Ali A. Mehdirad and Richard Lee

*Address all correspondence to: kpatel74@slu.edu

Center for Comprehensive Cardiovascular Care, Saint Louis University School of Medicine, St Louis, MO, USA

References

[1] Fuster V, Ryden LE, Cannom DS, et al. ACC/AHA/ESC 2006 guidelines for the management of patients with atrial fibrillation. Circulation. 2006; 114:e257–e354.

[2] Hart RG, Benavente O, McBride R, Pearce LA. Antithrombotic therapy to prevent stroke in patients with atrial fibrillation: a meta-analysis. Ann Intern Med. 1999; 131:492–501.

[3] Agarwal S, Hachamovitch R, Menon V. Current trial-associated outcomes with warfarin in prevention of stroke in patients with non-valvular atrial fibrillation: a meta-analysis. Arch Intern Med. 2012; 172:623–631.

[4] You JJ, Singer DE, Howard PA, et al. Antithrombotic therapy for atrial fibrillation. Chest. 2012; 141(2_suppl):e531S–e575S.doi:10.1378/chest.11-2304.

[5] Coppens M, Eikelboom JW, Hart RG, Yusuf S, Lip GY, Dorian P, et al. The CHA2DS2-VASc score identifies those patients with atrial fibrillation and a CHADS2 score of 1 who are unlikely to benefit from oral anticoagulant therapy. Eur Heart J. 2013; 34:170–176

[6] Friberg L, Hammar N, Ringh M, Pettersson H, Rosenqvist M. Stroke prophylaxis in atrial fibrillation: who gets it and who does not? (SCAF-study). Eur Heart J. 2006; 27(16): 1954–1964.

[7] Gladstone D, Bui E, Fang J, Laupacis A, Lindsay MP, Tu JV, et al. Potentially preventable strokes in high-risk patients with atrial fibrillation who are not adequately anticoagulated. Stroke. 2009; 40:235–240.

[8] Dabigatran (Pradaxa Dabigatran tablets) prescribing information [package insert]. Ridgefield, CT: Boehringer Ingelheim Pharmaceuticals, Inc.; 2010.

[9] Rivaroxaban (Xarelto Rivaroxaban tablets) prescribing information [package insert]. Titusville, NJ: Janssen Pharmaceuticals Inc.; 2011.

[10] U.S. Food and Drug Administration. Daiichi Sankyo briefing document for the cardiovascular and renal drugs advisory committee on Edoxaban. Available at: http://www.fda.gov/downloads/AdvisoryCommittees/CommitteesMeetingMaterials/

Drugs/CardiovascularandRenalDrugsAdvisoryCommittee/UCM420704.pdf. Accessed December 20, 2015.

[11] U.S. Food and Drug Administration. Boehringer Ingelheim advisory committee briefing document for Dabigatran. Available at: http://www.fda.gov/downloads/advisorycommittees/committeemeetingmaterials/drugs/cardiovascularandrenal-drugsadvisorycommittee/ucm226009.pdf. Accessed December 20, 2015.

[12] U.S. Food and Drug Administration. Johnson & Johnson briefing document for the cardiovascular and renal drugs advisory committee on Rivaroxaban. Available at: http://www.fda.gov/downloads/advisorycommittees/committeesmeetingmaterials/drugs/cardiovascularandrenaldrugsadvisorycommittee/ucm270796.pdf. Accessed December 20, 2015.

[13] Apixaban (Eliquis Apixaban tablets) prescribing information [package insert]. Princeton, NJ: Bristol-Myers Squibb Co.; 2012.

[14] Giugliano RP, et al. (2013). Edoxaban versus warfarin in patients with atrial fibrillation. N Engl J Med. 369(22): 2093-2104.

[15] Büller HR, Décousus H, Grosso MA, Mercuri M, Middeldorp S, Prins MH, et al. Edoxaban versus warfarin for the treatment of symptomatic venous thromboembolism. N Engl J Med. 2013; 369:1406–1415.

[16] Edoxaban (Savaysa Edoxaban tablets) prescribing information [package insert]. Parsippany, NJ: Daiichi Sankyo, Inc.; 2011.

[17] Granger CB, Alexander JH, McMurray JJ, et al. Apixaban versus warfarin in patients with atrial fibrillation. N Engl J Med. 2011; 365:981–992.

[18] Connolly SJ, Ezekowitz MD, Yusuf S, et al. Dabigatran versus warfarin in patients with atrial fibrillation. N Engl J Med. 2009; 361:1139–1151.

[19] Patel MR, Mahaffey KW, Garg J, et al. Rivaroxaban versus warfarin in non-valvular atrial fibrillation. N Engl J Med. 2011; 365:883–891.

[20] Rosendaal FR, Cannegieter SC, van der Meer FJ, Briet E. A method to determine the optimal intensity of oral anticoagulant therapy. Thromb Haemost. 1993; 69:236–239.

[21] Wallentin L, Yusuf S, Ezekowitz MD, et al. Efficacy and safety of Dabigatran compared with warfarin at different levels of international normalized ratio control for stroke prevention in atrial fibrillation: an analysis of the RE-LY trial. Lancet. 2010; 376:975–983.

[22] Uchino K, Hernandez AV. Dabigatran association with higher risk of acute coronary events: meta-analysis of non-inferiority randomized controlled trials. Arch Intern Med. 2012; 172(5):397–402

[23] Douxfils J, Buckinx F, Mullier F, et al. Dabigatran etexilate and risk of myocardial infarction, other cardiovascular events, major bleeding, and all-cause mortality: a

http://dx.doi.org/10.5772/64440

systematic review and meta-analysis of randomized controlled trials. J Am Heart Assoc. 2014; 3(3):e000515

[24] FDA Drug Safety Communication: FDA Study of Medicare Patients Finds Risks Lower for Stroke and Death but Higher for Gastrointestinal Bleeding with Pradaxa (Dabigatran) Compared to Warfarin. *FDA Drug Safety Communication: FDA Study of Medicare Patients Finds Risks Lower for Stroke and Death but Higher for Gastrointestinal Bleeding with Pradaxa (Dabigatran) Compared to Warfarin.* US Food and Drug Administration, Nov. 11, 2012. Web. May 20, 2016.

Chapter 7

Non–Vitamin K Antagonist Oral Anticoagulants, Clinical Use, Real-World Data, and Reversal of Anticoagulant Effect

Özcan Başaran, Volkan Doğan, Ibrahim Altun and
Murat Biteker

Additional information is available at the end of the chapter

http://dx.doi.org/10.5772/64464

Abstract

Atrial fibrillation (AF) is the most common sustained cardiac arrhythmia in clinical practice and is associated with a higher risk of thromboembolic events. CHA_2DS_2VASc score enables identification of those patients with AF who will most benefit from anticoagulation therapy and low-risk patients with AF who do not need any antithrombotic therapy. Antithrombotic drugs especially oral anticoagulants (OACs) are the mainstay of therapy to prevent stroke in patients with AF. Although vitamin K antagonists (VKAs) were the only available drugs for decades, numerous non–vitamin K antagonist oral anticoagulants (NOACs) have been developed and marketed for stroke prevention in recent years. The risk of stroke was reported to decline up to 68 % with OAC therapy, associated with good anticoagulation control with VKAs, assessed by time in therapeutic range (TTR). In low TTR values, VKAs were found to be associated with severe complications, and a minimum TTR of 58 % should be achieved to expect a net benefit from being on OAC therapy. Narrow therapeutic index, drug-drug interactions, and the need for close monitoring are the main disadvantages of VKAs, and management of patients have dramatically improved after the introduction of NOACs. NOACs have a more predictable anticoagulant affect which allows a fixed-dose regimen. The efficacy and safety of NOACs have been shown not only in large randomized controlled clinical trials but also in observational studies. The main advantages of NOACS such as "fixed-dose regimen" and "no need for regular anticoagulant therapy monitoring" may also be the Achilles heel of the use of these agents. Fixed-dose regimen may not be appropriate for elderly, for patients with chronic kidney disease, and for patients using interacting drugs. Adherence to NOAC therapy is another concern as it may be as low as 50 % in the chronic use of cardiovascular drugs, especially if the drug has no apparent affect to the patient. Thus, appropriate use of

OACs among non-valvular AF (NVAF) patients is essential for stroke prophylaxis. We intended to review the use of OAC therapy among (NVAF) patients.

Keywords: Oral anticoagulants, Atrial fibrillation, Stroke prophylaxis

1. Introduction

Atrial fibrillation (AF) is the most common sustained cardiac arrhythmia in clinical practice and is associated with a higher risk of thromboembolic events [1]. The most devastating complication of AF is ischemic stroke. AF is the most frequent cause of cardioembolic stroke and nearly 20 % of all stroke events. Cardioembolic stroke has a greater morbidity and mortality comparing other stroke subtypes. Nevertheless, oral anticoagulant (OAC) drugs offer an effective stroke prevention strategy [2]. Recent guidelines recommend to start an OAC drug for patients who have AF and high risk of stroke assessed by stroke risk schemes [3]. The most recommended risk scheme is known by the acronym CHA_2DS_2VASc (congestive heart failure, hypertension, age ≥75, diabetes, stroke history, vascular disease, ages 65–74, and sex), and patients with a score ≥2 should be anticoagulated. The discovery and development of anticoagulants are some of the most interesting in pharmaceutical history and started with the discovery of heparin in 1916 (**Figure 1**). Studies on anticoagulant drugs led to the commercialization of dicoumarol in 1941, and efforts to develop an effective rodenticide resulted in synthesis of warfarin (Wisconsin Alumni Research Foundation), which was approved for medical use in 1954. For decades, vitamin K antagonists (VKAs) were the only available oral anticoagulants. The risk of stroke was reported to decline up to 68 % with OAC therapy, associated with good anticoagulation control with VKAs, assessed by time in therapeutic range (TTR). In low TTR values VKAs were found to be associated with severe complications, and a minimum TTR of 58 % should be achieved to expect a net benefit from being on OAC therapy [4]. The use of VKAs can also be challenging due to narrow therapeutic index, drug-drug interactions, and the need for close monitoring. Over the last years, non–vitamin K antagonist oral anticoagulants (NOACs) have been developed, including direct thrombin inhibitors (dabigatran) and factor Xa inhibitors (rivarox-

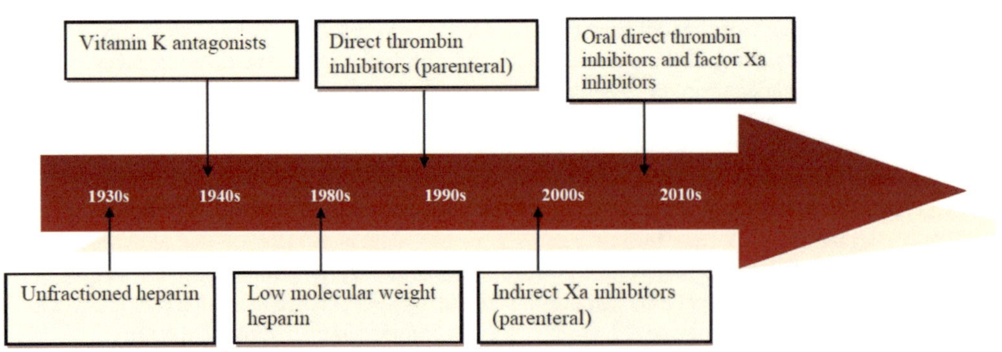

Figure 1. Developmental history of anticoagulants.

http://dx.doi.org/10.5772/64464

aban, apixaban, and edoxaban) which have a more predictable anticoagulant affect allowing a fixed-dose regimen. Their therapeutic use for prevention of cardioembolic complications was validated in large phase III trials, demonstrating their non-inferiority and even superiority, in some cases, to warfarin [5–8]. Therefore, the use of NOACs is currently recommended by guidelines, along with VKAs, for stroke prevention in patients with non-valvular atrial fibrillation (NVAF). The risk of hemorrhage should also be assessed prior to starting an OAC drug. One of the validated risk scores is hypertension, renal or liver failure, stroke history, bleeding history, labile international normalized ratio (INR), age > 65 years, drugs predisposing to bleeding, and alcohol use (HAS-BLED). Bleeding risk assessment with HAS-BLED should not be used as an excuse not to prescribe OAC but rather to highlight those patients in whom caution with such treatment and regular review is warranted. Both VKA and NOACs have specific targets in the coagulation cascade (**Figure 2**). The INR is widely used for the measurement of anticoagulant effect of VKAs. However, the anticoagulant effect of NOACs cannot be measured with routine coagulation assays. While activated partial thromboplastin time (aPTT) is elevated in patients taking dabigatran and edoxaban, it is not correlated with the dose of the drug. Ecarin-clotting time (ECT), thrombin time (TT), and dilute thrombin time (dTT) assays

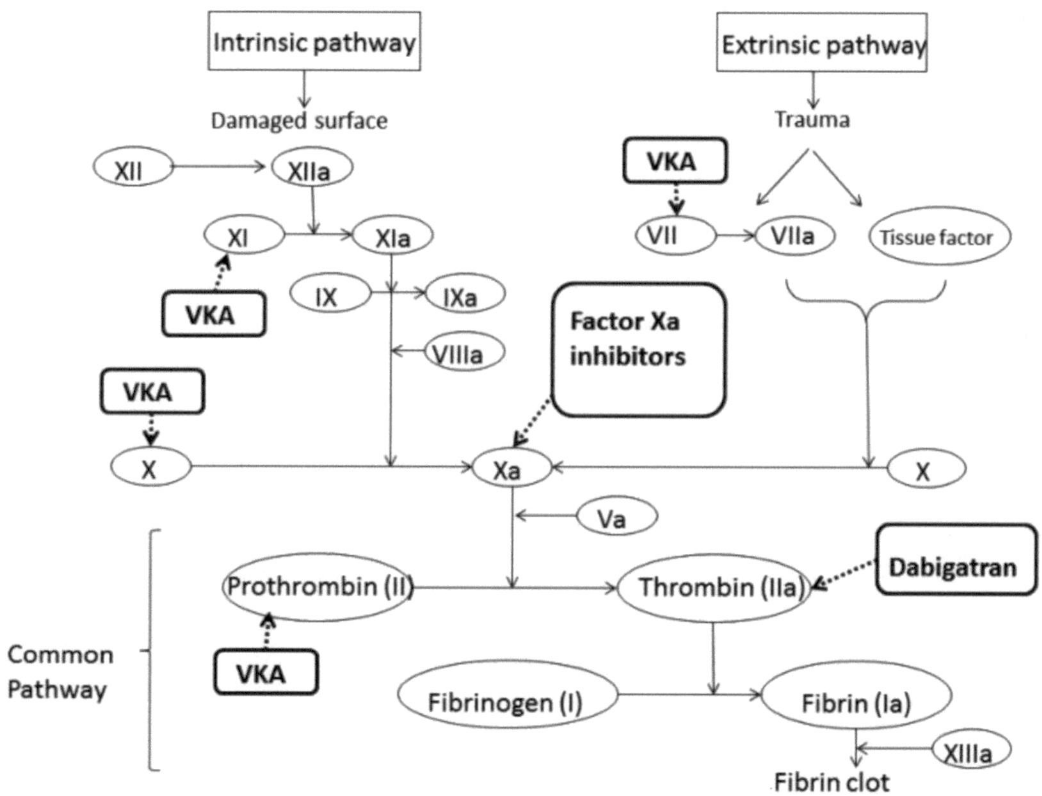

Figure 2. The coagulation cascade. VKA, vitamin K antagonist.

might be used for dabigatran's anticoagulant effect and anti-factor Xa assays for rivaroxaban and apixaban. However, these assays are not commercially available that restricts their use in most institutions. Although NOACs have clear advantages comparing warfarin, it may not be convenient for some patients. They were not studied in patients with severe renal failure (estimated glomerular filtration rate (GFR) <30 mL/min), and a dose reduction is recommended for patients with moderate renal failure (GFR: 30–50 mL/min). The use of NOACs in patients with mechanical heart valves is contraindicated. The RE-ALIGN (randomized, phase II study to evaluate the safety and pharmacokinetics of oral dabigatran etexilate in patients after heart valve replacement) study showed that dabigatran was neither effective nor safe in patients with mechanical heart valves [8]. However, it was safe and effective in other types of valvular diseases such as mitral regurgitation, aortic regurgitation, aortic stenosis, tricuspid regurgitation, and mild mitral stenosis [9]. Thus the term "valvular AF" defines patients with mechanical heart valves and patients with mitral stenosis (mostly rheumatic) [10]. In this chapter, we will review the clinical use, real-world data, and reversal of anticoagulant effect of NOACs for stroke prevention in patients with NVAF as well as discuss the limitations of the new agents.

2. Direct thrombin inhibitors

Direct thrombin inhibitors act by inhibiting thrombin which converts fibrinogen to fibrin and activates platelets (**Figure 2**). Ximelagatran was the first-studied direct thrombin inhibitor for stroke prophylaxis in NVAF patients, but it was withdrawn from market because of safety concerns about hepatotoxicity.

2.1. Dabigatran

Dabigatran was the first-introduced NOAC into clinical practice. It was predominantly eliminated by kidneys; thus, a dose reduction was proposed for patients with renal failure [3]. The European Medical Agency (EMA) has approved two doses (110 and 150 mg) of dabigatran with a recommendation of dose reduction in older patients with renal failure. However, Food and Drug Administration (FDA) did not approve the 110 mg bid and approved 75 mg bid for patients with renal failure. FDA recommended the higher dose (150 mg bid) for most of the patients. Though it remains a controversial issue, FDA did not change its recommendations after a mini-sentinel [11]; however, a post hoc analysis of RE-LY trial showed better outcomes if European label was used [12]. Nevertheless, with the available data for both doses, dabigatran is an attractive alternative to warfarin in patients with NVAF. A meta-analysis of real-world data also showed similar efficacy compared to warfarin with less intracranial bleeding [13]. The authors concluded dabigatran should be used cautiously in older patients with a history of gastrointestinal bleeding.

Although dabigatran was well tolerated, prevalence of dyspepsia was increased compared to warfarin (11.8 % with 110 mg bid, 11.3 % with 150 mg bid, 5.8 % with warfarin). This side effect has been attributed to tartaric acid component in dabigatran etexilate capsule [14]. Although dabigatran has lower rates of drug-drug interaction, it has significant interaction with p-glycoprotein inhibitors (e.g., ketoconazole, amiodarone, verapamil) and inducers (rifampin). A dose reduction was proposed for patients taking concomitant verapamil.

3. Factor Xa inhibitors

Factor Xa has an important role in the coagulation cascade (**Figure 2**). Currently there are three approved factor Xa inhibitors—rivaroxaban, apixaban, and edoxaban—and one under investigation betrixaban.

3.1. Rivaroxaban

Rivaroxaban was the first-approved factor Xa inhibitor for stroke prophylaxis in NVAF. Rivaroxaban 15 mg od was given for patients with creatinine clearance 30–50 mL/min. It was found as effective as warfarin for stroke or systemic embolism prevention without an increase in major bleeding [7]. In addition, it was associated with less intracranial bleeding. Real-world analysis of rivaroxaban also revealed comparable bleeding rates with phase III trial with a significant heterogeneity in bleeding rates across studies [15]. A real-world analysis of rivaroxaban showed similar results comparing warfarin for safety and efficacy; however, venous thromboembolism (VTE) events were fewer in rivaroxaban patients [16]. Another real-world analysis showed that rivaroxaban may even be better in terms of hemorrhagic complications or at least as safe as warfarin [17]. Coleman et al. showed that rivaroxaban may be better for stroke prophylaxis in a German medical record study [18]. In conclusion, rivaroxaban was shown to be as effective and safe as warfarin in real-world data.

3.2. Apixaban

Apixaban is a factor Xa inhibitor that has been approved for stroke prophylaxis in patients with NVAF. The risk of gastrointestinal bleeding was comparable between apixaban and warfarin, and apixaban showed a reduction in mortality rates [6]. Apixaban was also evaluated in patients who could not take warfarin in apixaban versus acetylsalicylic acid to prevent stroke (AVERROES) trial [19]. Apixaban was more effective and as safe as aspirin in stroke prophylaxis; thus, the study was prematurely terminated because of clear advantage of apixaban. The benefits of apixaban were consistent regardless of age with a greater absolute risk reduction in the elderly [20].

3.3. Edoxaban

Edoxaban is a factor Xa inhibitor that has been approved for stroke prophylaxis recently. It has been tested in two different doses (30 and 60 mg) against warfarin [5]. The high dose of edoxaban was associated with a trend toward better efficacy versus warfarin for stroke and systemic embolism prophylaxis. A real-world modeling analysis also showed edoxaban 60 mg od might be superior to warfarin and 30 mg od dose [21]. The efficacy of edoxaban was decreased in patients with a creatine clearance <95 mL/min. Thus it is not recommended in these patients.

3.4. Betrixaban

Betrixaban is a factor Xa inhibitor with minimal renal excretion and a long half-life. It has minimal hepatic metabolism. Thus it could be used for patients with renal and hepatic impairment. The anticoagulant effect and safety of betrixaban were compared against warfarin in NVAF patients in a phase II study (EXPLORE-Xa) [22]. Betrixaban was well tolerated, and bleeding was lowest in betrixaban 40 mg group compared warfarin or betrixaban 60–80 mg. The study was primarily designed to assess safety of betrixaban, and it does not provide an information for the efficacy. The pharmacometric modeling suggests that 80 mg daily betrixaban has comparable anticoagulant effect to warfarin. The ongoing phase III trial (APEX) is currently investigating the protective effect of betrixaban in venous thromboembolism (VTE) against enoxaparin in acute medically ill patients. The topline results of the study showed betrixaban given once daily at a dose of 80 mg for 35–47 days was more effective than injectable enoxaparin given at a dose of 40 mg for 6–14 days [23]. There was no increase in major bleeding rates.

4. Comparison of real-world data and phase III trials

Large phase III trials showed a comparable effect and better safety profile of NOACs for stroke thromboprophylaxis. However, these studies included highly selected patients without severe comorbidities with strict follow-up procedures. In addition all the patients in these trials were OAC indicated. However, observational studies showed OAC use was 60–80 % in real-world settings [24–27]. Another concern regarding OAC therapy is the appropriate use. Inappropriate use might be up to 87 % in warfarin and 47 % in NOACs [28, 29]. The efficacy and safety of NOACs were confirmed in observational studies. Danish registry compared the safety and efficacy of dabigatran against warfarin [30]. Both 110 and 150 mg bid doses of dabigatran were as effective as warfarin for stroke prophylaxis, and 110 mg bid but not 150 mg bid was associated with lower rates of gastrointestinal bleeding. A recent meta-analysis also showed similar stroke rates with dabigatran comparing warfarin and lower intracranial bleeding with an elevated risk for gastrointestinal bleeding [24]. Xarelto® on prevention of stroke and non-central nervous system systemic embolism in patients with non-valvular atrial fibrillation (XANTUS) trial with rivaroxaban showed better efficacy and safety profile in a real-world dataset [31]. A propensity score-matched study also showed the efficacy and safety of rivaroxaban in real-world data [32]. These observations showed NOACs are safe and effective treatment options for stroke prevention in NVAF patients. However, a recent real-world database study from the USA revealed a 4.4-fold increase in the use of reduced dose of apixaban comparing ARISTOTLE trial [33].

5. Reversal agents

One of the main difficulties with NOACs is the lack of specific reversal agents. Despite the lower rates of hemorrhage with NOACs comparing warfarin, a hemorrhagic complication that needs medical support may occur with NOACs. While a minor bleeding might be solved with supportive care, specific medications should be used for major bleedings. Perioperative management for patients on NOAC may also be challenging especially in emergency situations. Activated charcoal should be administered if the drug has recently been taken. Hemodialysis is an option for patients on dabigatran. Tranexamic acid and aminocaproic acid are also nonspecific agents that can be used to control bleeding. Fresh frozen plasma is not an option; however, prothrombin plasma concentrates (PCC) especially four-factor PCC are more useful. However, there has been an unmet need for specific reversal agents until idarucizumab's FDA approval. Idarucizumab is a monoclonal antibody that was approved for reversal of dabigatran's anticoagulant effect. Andexanet alfa is a specific antidote of factor Xa inhibitors, and ciraparantag is a universal reversal agent.

5.1. Idarucizumab

Idarucizumab is a monoclonal antibody fragment that specifically binds to dabigatran and antagonizes its effect at a 1:1 ratio. Its half-life is 45 min and thus it may require repeat infusion. The effect of idarucizumab was shown by measuring dTT and ECT which are specific for dabigatran activity. The efficacy and safety of idarucizumab were evaluated in RE-VERSE AD (a study of the reversal effects of idarucizumab on active dabigatran) phase III trial, and a 5 g intravenous infusion was found safe and effective [34]. In 35 patients with major bleeding, hemostasis was restored at a median of 11.4 h, and in 36 patients who underwent urgent procedure, normal hemostasis was reported in 33, mildly abnormal in 2, and moderately abnormal in 1 patient. Idarucizumab was approved by FDA for the reversal of dabigatran's anticoagulant effect. It does not have prolonged effect, and dabigatran can be restarted after 24 h.

5.2. Andexanet alfa

Andexanet alfa is a recombinant factor Xa inhibitor antidote. It specifically binds to factor Xa inhibitors thus reduces their unbound concentrations. It has been studied in animal and human studies and reversed anticoagulant effect of rivaroxaban, apixaban, and edoxaban [35, 36]. The effect of andexanet alfa disappears in the absence of a maintenance infusion. Consistent with the half-life of andexanet alfa, the anticoagulant effect reversal was comparable with placebo after 2 h cessation of infusion. Levels of D-dimer and prothrombin fragments 1 and 2 were elevated in patients receiving andexanet alfa; however, this was not associated with clinical thrombotic events [36]. Andexanet alfa is a potential universal antidote for factor Xa inhibitors.

5.3. Ciraparantag

Ciraparantag is a small molecule that binds unfractionated and low-molecular-weight heparin. It binds to endogenous targets of anticoagulants that prevent their anticoagulant effect. It also binds to dabigatran and factor Xa inhibitors; thus, it has a wide range of action. The first human study with this drug reported effective and safe reversal of anticoagulant effect of edoxaban within 10–30 min [37]. Ciraparantag is a promising universal reversal agent of anticoagulant effect.

6. Conclusion

The risk of ischemic stroke is increased in patients with AF. Recent guidelines for the evaluation of AF recommend OAC therapy for AF patients who had moderate to high risk of stroke. Although NOACs have clear advantages over warfarin, there are some concerns such as the lack of specific antidote, older patients, lower creatinine clearance, risk of gastrointestinal hemorrhage, and cost. Specific antidotes are under development—idarucizumab has already been approved—and lower doses of the drugs might be a solution for high-bleeding-risk-group patients. The phase III trials and real-world data indicated NOACs were as safe and effective as warfarin, while some studies showed better net clinical benefit with NOACs. The introduction of NOACs has led to an improvement in the management of patients with NVAF; however, there is need for great effort for the optimization of stroke prevention strategies in AF.

Author details

Özcan Başaran*, Volkan Doğan, Ibrahim Altun and Murat Biteker

*Address all correspondence to: basaran_ozcan@yahoo.com

Department of Cardiology, Faculty of Medicine, Muğla Sıtkı Koçman University, Muğla, Turkey

References

[1] Go AS, Hylek EM, Phillips KA, Chang Y, Henault LE, Selby JV, et al. Prevalence of diagnosed atrial fibrillation in adults. JAMA [Internet]; 2001 May 9 [cited 2016 Apr 6]; 285(18):2370. Available from: http://jama.jamanetwork.com/article.aspx?doi=10.1001/jama.285.18.2370

[2] Hart RG, Pearce LA, Aguilar MI. Meta-analysis: antithrombotic therapy to prevent stroke in patients who have nonvalvular atrial fibrillation. Ann Intern Med [Internet]. 2007 Jun 19 [cited 2016 Apr 6];146(12):857–67. Available from: http://www.ncbi.nlm.nih.gov/pubmed/17577005

[3] Camm AJ, Lip GYH, De Caterina R, Savelieva I, Atar D, Hohnloser SH, et al. 2012 focused update of the ESC Guidelines for the management of atrial fibrillation. Eur

Heart J [Internet]. 2012;33(21):2719–47. Available from: http://eurheartj.oxfordjournals.org/content/33/21/2719.abstract

[4] Connolly SJ, Pogue J, Eikelboom J, Flaker G, Commerford P, Franzosi MG, et al. Benefit of oral anticoagulant over antiplatelet therapy in atrial fibrillation depends on the quality of international normalized ratio control achieved by centers and countries as measured by time in therapeutic range. Circulation [Internet]. 2008 Nov 11 [cited 2016 Apr 19];118(20):2029–37. Available from: http://circ.ahajournals.org/cgi/doi/10.1161/CIRCULATIONAHA.107.750000

[5] Giugliano RP, Ruff CT, Braunwald E, Murphy SA, Wiviott SD, Halperin JL, et al. Edoxaban versus warfarin in patients with atrial fibrillation. N Engl J Med [Internet]. 2013;369:2093–104. Available from: http://www.ncbi.nlm.nih.gov/pubmed/24251359

[6] Granger CB, Alexander JH, McMurray JJ V, Lopes RD, Hylek EM, Hanna M, et al. Apixaban versus warfarin in patients with atrial fibrillation. N Engl J Med [Internet]. 2011;365(11):981–92. Available from: http://www.ncbi.nlm.nih.gov/pubmed/21870978

[7] Patel MR, Mahaffey KW, Garg J, Pan G, Singer DE, Hacke W, et al. Rivaroxaban versus warfarin in nonvalvular atrial fibrillation. N Engl J Med [Internet]. 2011;365(10):883–91. Available from: http://www.ncbi.nlm.nih.gov/pubmed/21830957

[8] Eikelboom JW, Connolly SJ, Brueckmann M, Granger CB, Kappetein AP, Mack MJ, et al. Dabigatran versus warfarin in patients with mechanical heart valves. N Engl J Med [Internet]. 2013 Sep 26 [cited 2016 Apr 16];369(13):1206–14. Available from: http://www.nejm.org/doi/abs/10.1056/NEJMoa1300615

[9] Ezekowitz MD, Parise H, Nagarakanti R, Noack H, Brueckmann M, Clemens A, et al. comparison of dabigatran versus warfarin in patients with atrial fibrillation and valvular heart disease: the re-ly® trial. J Am Coll Cardiol [Internet]; 2014 Apr [cited 2016 Apr 16];63(12):A325. Available from: http://linkinghub.elsevier.com/retrieve/pii/S0735109714603259

[10] Başaran Ö, Doğan V, Şahin C, Biteker M, Noseworthy PA, Yao X, et al. Non-vitamin K antagonist oral anticoagulants in valvular atrial fibrillation. Int J Cardiol [Internet]; 2016 Jun [cited 2016 Apr 17];212:357. Available from: http://linkinghub.elsevier.com/retrieve/pii/S0167527316305502

[11] Southworth MR, Reichman ME, Unger EF. Dabigatran and postmarketing reports of bleeding. N Engl J Med [Internet]. 2013 Apr 4 [cited 2016 May 9];368(14):1272–4. Available from: http://www.ncbi.nlm.nih.gov/pubmed/23484796

[12] Lip GYH, Clemens A, Noack H, Ferreira J, Connolly SJ, Yusuf S. Patient outcomes using the European label for dabigatran. A post-hoc analysis from the RE-LY database. Thromb Haemost [Internet]. 2014 May 5 [cited 2016 Apr 6];111(5):933–42. Available from: http://www.ncbi.nlm.nih.gov/pubmed/24326736

[13] Romanelli RJ, Nolting L, Dolginsky M, Kym E, Orrico KB. Dabigatran versus warfarin for atrial fibrillation in real-world clinical practice: a systematic review and meta-

analysis. Circ Cardiovasc Qual Outcomes [Internet]. 2016 Mar [cited 2016 May 9];9(2): 126–34. Available from: http://www.ncbi.nlm.nih.gov/pubmed/26812933

[14] Connolly SJ, Ezekowitz MD, Yusuf S, Eikelboom J, Oldgren J, Parekh A, et al. Dabigatran versus warfarin in patients with atrial fibrillation. N Engl J Med [Internet]. 2009;361(12):1139–51. Available from: http://www.ncbi.nlm.nih.gov/pubmed/19717844

[15] Weeda ER, White CM, Peacock WF, Coleman CI. Rates of major bleeding with rivaroxaban in real-world studies of nonvalvular atrial fibrillation patients: a meta-analysis. Curr Med Res Opin [Internet]. 2016 Mar 16 [cited 2016 May 18];1–4. Available from: http://www.tandfonline.com/doi/full/10.1185/03007995.2016.1161610

[16] Laliberté F, Cloutier M, Nelson WW, Coleman CI, Pilon D, Olson WH, et al. Real-world comparative effectiveness and safety of rivaroxaban and warfarin in nonvalvular atrial fibrillation patients. Curr Med Res Opin [Internet]. 2014 Jul [cited 2016 May 18];30(7): 1317–25. Available from: http://www.ncbi.nlm.nih.gov/pubmed/24650301

[17] Beyer-Westendorf J, Förster K, Pannach S, Ebertz F, Gelbricht V, Thieme C, et al. Rates, management, and outcome of rivaroxaban bleeding in daily care: results from the Dresden NOAC registry. Blood [Internet]. 2014 Aug 7 [cited 2016 May 18];124(6):955–62. Available from: http://www.ncbi.nlm.nih.gov/pubmed/24859362

[18] Coleman CI, Antz M, Ehlken B, Evers T, Patel MR, Mahaffey KW, et al. REal-LIfe Evidence of stroke prevention in patients with atrial Fibrillation—the RELIEF study. Int J Cardiol [Internet]; 2016 Jan [cited 2016 May 18];203:882–4. Available from: http://linkinghub.elsevier.com/retrieve/pii/S0167527315304769

[19] Connolly SJ, Eikelboom J, Joyner C, Diener H-C, Hart R, Golitsyn S, et al. Apixaban in Patients with Atrial Fibrillation. N Engl J Med [Internet]. 2011 Mar 3 [cited 2016 Apr 19];364(9):806–17. Available from: http://www.nejm.org/doi/abs/10.1056/NEJMoa1007432

[20] Halvorsen S, Atar D, Yang H, De Caterina R, Erol C, Garcia D, et al. Efficacy and safety of apixaban compared with warfarin according to age for stroke prevention in atrial fibrillation: observations from the ARISTOTLE trial. Eur Heart J. 2014 Jul 21;35(28): 1864–72

[21] Blann AD, Banerjee A, Lane DA, Torp-Pedersen C, Lip GYH. Net clinical benefit of edoxaban versus no treatment in a "real world" atrial fibrillation population: a modelling analysis based on a nationwide cohort study. Int J Cardiol [Internet]. 2015 Dec 15 [cited 2016 May 18];201:693–8. Available from: http://www.ncbi.nlm.nih.gov/pubmed/26379097

[22] Connolly SJ, Eikelboom J, Dorian P, Hohnloser SH, Gretler DD, Sinha U, et al. Betrixaban compared with warfarin in patients with atrial fibrillation: results of a phase 2, randomized, dose-ranging study (Explore-Xa). Eur Heart J [Internet]. 2013 May [cited

2016 Apr 14];34(20):1498–505. Available from: http://www.ncbi.nlm.nih.gov/pubmed/23487517

[23] Portola Pharmaceuticals Announces Topline Results from Phase 3 APEX Trial of Betrixaban for Prevention of Blood Clots in Acute Medically Ill Patients [Internet]. 2016. Available from: http://investors.portola.com/phoenix.zhtml?c=198136&p=irol-newsroomArticle&ID=2150685

[24] Romanelli RJ, Nolting L, Dolginsky M, Kym E, Orrico KB. Dabigatran versus warfarin for atrial fibrillation in real-world clinical practice. Circ Cardiovasc Qual Outcomes [Internet]. 2016 Mar [cited 2016 Apr 19];9(2):126–34. Available from: http://circoutcomes.ahajournals.org/lookup/doi/10.1161/CIRCOUTCOMES.115.002369

[25] Fumagalli S, Said SAM, Laroche C, Gabbai D, Marchionni N, Boriani G, et al. Age-related differences in presentation, treatment, and outcome of patients with atrial fibrillation in Europe. JACC Clin Electrophysiol [Internet]. 2015 Aug [cited 2016 Feb 3]; 1(4):326–34. Available from: http://www.sciencedirect.com/science/article/pii/S2405500X15000936

[26] Huisman M V, Rothman KJ, Paquette M, Teutsch C, Diener HC, Dubner SJ, et al. Antithrombotic treatment patterns in patients with newly diagnosed nonvalvular atrial fibrillation: the GLORIA-AF Registry, Phase II. Am J Med [Internet]. 2015 Dec [cited 2015 Dec 14];128(12):1306–13.e1. Available from: http://www.ncbi.nlm.nih.gov/pubmed/26239094

[27] Basaran O. ReAl-life Multicenter Survey Evaluating Stroke prevention strategies in non-valvular atrial fibrillation (RAMSES study). Anatol J Cardiol [Internet]. 2016 [cited 2016 Apr 19]; Available from: http://www.journalagent.com/anatoljcardiol/pdfs/AJC-04127-ORIGINAL_INVESTIGATION-BASARAN.pdf

[28] Basaran O, Filiz Basaran N, Cekic EG, Altun I, Dogan V, Mert GO, et al. PRescriptiOn PattERns of Oral Anticoagulants in Nonvalvular Atrial Fibrillation (PROPER study). Clin Appl Thromb Hemost [Internet]. 2015 Oct 30 [cited 2016 Apr 19]; Available from: http://www.ncbi.nlm.nih.gov/pubmed/26519049

[29] Bell AD, Gross P, Heffernan M, Deschaintre Y, Roux J-F, Purdham DM, et al. Appropriate use of antithrombotic medication in canadian patients with nonvalvular atrial fibrillation. Am J Cardiol [Internet]. 2016 Apr 1 [cited 2016 Apr 19];117(7):1107–11. Available from: http://www.ncbi.nlm.nih.gov/pubmed/26879070

[30] Larsen TB, Rasmussen LH, Skjøth F, Due KM, Callréus T, Rosenzweig M, et al. Efficacy and safety of dabigatran etexilate and warfarin in `real-world' patients with atrial fibrillation: a prospective nationwide cohort study. J Am Coll Cardiol [Internet]. 2013 Jun 4 [cited 2016 Apr 18];61(22):2264–73. Available from: http://www.ncbi.nlm.nih.gov/pubmed/23562920

[31] Camm AJ, Amarenco P, Haas S, Hess S, Kirchhof P, Kuhls S, et al. XANTUS: a real-world, prospective, observational study of patients treated with rivaroxaban for stroke

prevention in atrial fibrillation. Eur Heart J [Internet]. The Oxford University Press; 2016 Apr 7 [cited 2016 Apr 19];37(14):1145–53. Available from: http://www.ncbi.nlm.nih.gov/pubmed/26330425

[32] Laliberté F, Cloutier M, Nelson WW, Coleman CI, Pilon D, Olson WH, et al. Real-world comparative effectiveness and safety of rivaroxaban and warfarin in nonvalvular atrial fibrillation patients. Curr Med Res Opin [Internet]. 2014 Jul [cited 2016 Apr 19];30(7):1317–25. Available from: http://www.ncbi.nlm.nih.gov/pubmed/24650301

[33] Nguyen E, White CM, Patel MR, Fields LE, Peacock WF, Crivera C, et al. Doses of apixaban and rivaroxaban prescribed in real-world United States cardiology practices compared to registration trials. Curr Med Res Opin [Internet]. 2016 Apr 1 [cited 2016 May 12];1–3. Available from: http://www.ncbi.nlm.nih.gov/pubmed/27009372

[34] Pollack C V., Reilly PA, Eikelboom J, Glund S, Verhamme P, Bernstein RA, et al. Idarucizumab for dabigatran reversal. N Engl J Med [Internet]. 2015 Aug 6 [cited 2016 Apr 14];373(6):511–20. Available from: http://www.nejm.org/doi/abs/10.1056/NEJMoa1502000

[35] Lu G, DeGuzman FR, Hollenbach SJ, Karbarz MJ, Abe K, Lee G, et al. A specific antidote for reversal of anticoagulation by direct and indirect inhibitors of coagulation factor Xa. Nat Med [Internet]; 2013 Mar 3 [cited 2016 Apr 13];19(4):446–51. Available from: http://www.nature.com/doifinder/10.1038/nm.3102

[36] Siegal DM, Curnutte JT, Connolly SJ, Lu G, Conley PB, Wiens BL, et al. Andexanet alfa for the reversal of factor Xa inhibitor activity. N Engl J Med [Internet]. 2015 Dec 17 [cited 2016 Apr 13];373(25):2413–24. Available from: http://www.nejm.org/doi/abs/10.1056/NEJMoa1510991

[37] Ansell JE, Bakhru SH, Laulicht BE, Steiner SS, Grosso M, Brown K, et al. Use of PER977 to reverse the anticoagulant effect of edoxaban. N Engl J Med [Internet]. 2014 Nov 27 [cited 2016 Apr 13];371(22):2141–2. Available from: http://www.nejm.org/doi/abs/10.1056/NEJMc1411800